# THE HARRIET LANE HANDBOOK
## A Manual for Pediatric House Officers

# THE
# HARRIET LANE
# HANDBOOK
## A Manual for Pediatric House Officers

### SEVENTH EDITION

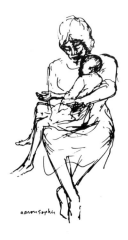

The Harriet Lane Service,
Children's Medical and Surgical Center
of the
Johns Hopkins Hospital

*Editor*
DENNIS L. HEADINGS, M.D.

YEAR BOOK MEDICAL PUBLISHERS, INC.
35 East Wacker Drive, Chicago

NOTICE

Every effort has been made to ensure that the drug dosage
schedules herein are accurate and in accord with the
standards accepted at the time of publication.  However,
as new research and experience broaden our knowledge,
changes in treatment and drug therapy occur.  Therefore,
the reader is advised to check the product information
sheet included in the package of each drug he plans to
administer to be certain that changes have not been made
in the recommended dose or in the contraindications.
This is of particular importance in regard to new or in-
frequently used drugs.

The Seventh Edition of the Harriet Lane Handbook comes at a very special time. The Harriet Lane Home for Invalid Children was torn down during the preparation of this manuscript as part of a rebuilding program of the Johns Hopkins Hospital. All of us who have been part of the Harriet Lane Service hope that the Pediatric Service and this Handbook will continue to remind us of our heritage of excellent patient care and child advocacy and encourage us to strive for continued achievements in these areas.

Over the past three years numerous suggestions have been incorporated. Some charts and procedures no longer used have been dropped, others altered for current use, and new information added. We hope that this book continues to reflect the needs of the pediatric house officers for whom it is primarily intended as a source of rapid information and reference. In keeping with this we have deleted the dosages of most oncology drugs because of the rapid growth of treatment protocols, but the most important side effects continue to be listed in the formulary.

I am indebted to the entire faculty for the numerous suggestions made both in writing and in person. Specifically I want to thank Dr. Dan Pieroni, Dr. Richard M. Heller, and Dr. Kate Morton for their help, and Dr. John Littlefield for his support of this new edition.

Special thanks go to the entire housestaff who made my year as Chief Resident a real pleasure. Dr. Kenneth Roberts, OPD Chief Resident, and the entire Senior Resident staff including Drs. James Allen, Michael Borzy, Stan Cohen, Alan Fleischman, Gary Gutcher, John Hayford, Marie McCormick, Kim Ritchey, Alberto Saenz, James Sutphen and Alan Zuckerman were most helpful throughout the year.

There were five Senior Residents who really served as contributing editors and deserve special credit. Dr. George Dover took on the massive job of revising the Formulary. Dr. Richard Cohn revised the Nephrology Section and contributed a great number of the new charts in the Therapeutics and Reference Sections. Dr. Alan Rogol revised the Endocrine Section; Dr. Frank Saulsbury re-edited the portion on Poisoning and Burns; and Dr. David Valle has redone the Metabolic Section of the Handbook. I owe them all a great deal for their help and friendship.

As before, none of this would have been possible without all those who have served and helped with previous Harriet Lane Handbooks. Thanks are due to previous editors, Drs. Henry Seidel, Harrison Spencer, William Friedman and Herbert Swick for material which has made its way from edition to edition. Two other previous editors to whom I owe special thanks are Dr. Robert Haslam and Dr. Jerry Winkelstein. I was fortunate to have both around not only for constant information and advice, but as friends and sources of inspiration. In this latter category I want to also pay tribute to Dr. William Zinkham and Dr. William MacLean who helped me get this done during my year as Chief Resident.

It was a real pleasure to work with Mr. William Keller and Mr. Ed Frank of the Yearbook Medical Publishers. I am most appreciative for their constant help and particularly their patience.

Finally, I want to thank three people without whom I could not have finished. Miss Kathy Morley, my secretary as OPD Chief Resident, got everything started back in early 1974; Miss Judy Safchuck was the efficient and cheerful typist for the manuscript; and Miss Susan Kinkel, my girl-Friday, served as general organizer, typist, proofreader and artist. I am most grateful to them all.

                                        Dennis L. Headings, M.D.
                                        Chief Resident
                                        Editor

Baltimore, 1975

TABLE OF CONTENTS

Preface

PART I - DIAGNOSTIC TESTS

## PART II - FORMULARY

## PART III - THERAPEUTIC DATA

## PART IV - REFERENCE DATA

PART I

DIAGNOSTIC TESTS

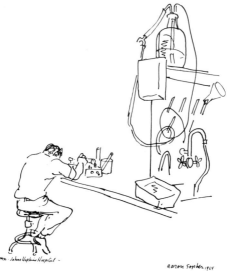

c mc. Johns Hopkins Hospital ~

aaron sopher 1964

P R O C E D U R E S

A.  OBTAINING BLOOD

1.  Capillary Blood

NOTE:  If obtained from extremity previously
heated to point of hyperemia, the capillary
blood is nearly identical to arterial blood
in acid-base properties.  Use right hand if
available.

a.  Heel and finger are convenient.  Avoid heel
    pad.
b.  Heat will produce local hyperemia.  Keep
    extremity used in dependent position.
c.  Use No. 11 Bard-Parker blade or deep lancet
    stab.
d.  Wipe away first drop of blood with dry
    sponge.  Alcohol used in sterilizing skin
    may produce hemolysis.
e.  Massage extremity but avoid squeezing
    finger or heel.

2.  External Jugular Puncture

a.  Wrap infant in mummified manner.
b.  Turn head to one side and extend.
c.  Prepare area carefully.
d.  Provoke child to cry in order to distend
    external jugular vein.
e.  "Scalp vein" needles with a syringe attached
    to the flexible tubing are easier and
    produce fewer infiltrations than straight
    needles.
f.  When needle is withdrawn, apply pressure
    and hold child upright.

3.  Femoral Puncture

NOTE:  Reported complication of septic arthritis demands careful and efficient skin antisep-
sis.

Ref:  Pediatrics 38:837, 1966.

NOTE:  Avoid femoral puncture in children that
are scheduled for cardiac catheterization.

a.  An assistant is needed to hold child
    securely.
b.  The assistant stands behind the infant,
    leans over the head and trunk and holds the
    legs in semi-frog position.  The arms of

the infant are held down by the assistant's
upper arms and elbows.
c.  Prepare area carefully as for blood culture.
d.  After locating the femoral pulse just below
the inguinal ligament, insert needle, aiming
slightly medial to the pulse beat.
e.  The needle is inserted slowly to a depth of
approximately 0.5 to 0.75 cm.
f.  While suction is exerted, needle is slowly
withdrawn until a small amount of blood
enters syringe.
g.  If flow ceases, needle is pushed deeper and
withdrawn as before.
h.  Both syringe and legs must be held station-
ary to insure drawing maximum amount of
blood.

4.  Internal Jugular Puncture

a.  Wrap infant securely in sheet.
b.  Place him on table and adjust position so
that head falls over the side.  With the
neck extended, head is turned slightly to
one side.  This makes the posterior margin
of the sternocleidomastoid muscle on the
opposite side stand out.
c.  Sterilize area.
d.  Needle is inserted just deep to and behind
posterior margin of sternocleidomastoid
muscle, approximately halfway between its
origin and insertion.  Needle is then
advanced under the muscle, parallel to skin
surface and in direction of suprasternal
notch, for a distance equal to width of
sternocleidomastoid.
e.  Needle is then slowly withdrawn while
keeping a negative pressure on syringe,
until point is reached at which blood enters
syringe.
f.  After blood is obtained, hold child upright
and apply pressure.

B.  BONE MARROW ASPIRATION

1.  General Comments and Warnings

a.  Bone marrow aspirations are always performed
with sterile surgical technique.
b.  Skin, soft tissue and periosteum are anes-
thetized with Procaine.
c.  Needle is inserted with boring motion and
steady but not excessive pressure.
d.  The classical description of a "give" when
the marrow cavity is entered is not only

             unreliable, but also indicates loss of control.

    e.  In children from birth to 6 months, the tibia is preferred site for aspiration.

    f.  Iliac crest is technically superior in children 6 months to 11 years of age.

    g.  No more than 0.2 ml of marrow should be aspirated, to minimize dilution with sinusoidal blood.

2. Iliac Marrow Technique

    a.  Patient lies on side, and iliac area is sterilized.

    b.  Anterior iliac crest is located at a point halfway between anterior and posterior spines.

    c.  The ilium is entered 2 cm below the outer lip perpendicular to the other table.

3. Tibial Marrow Technique

Best obtained from medial aspect of the head of the tibia, below medial condyle and tibial tuberosity. Needle inserted perpendicular to outer table.

4. Spinous Process

    a.  May be performed with patient in sitting position, leaning slightly forward.

    b.  Third or fourth lumbar vertebrae are preferred as these are likely to present broadest spinous process.

    c.  Needle is pushed through skin and inserted with rotary motion into the spinous process.

    d.  Instead of puncturing tip of spinous process directly, needle can be introduced into one side of it. It is then passed medially, entering the bone anteriorly to the tip, at a point where cortex is less thick.

5. Smear Technique

    a.  Eject marrow from syringe onto clean slide.

    b.  With another syringe and needle, aspirate excessive blood and plasma from marrow to concentrate marrow.

    c.  Using remaining marrow, make multiple smears in usual way.

C. SUPRAPUBIC ASPIRATION OF URINE

This technique of obtaining urine is most

advantageous in suspect urinary tract infections when clean catch urines are inconclusive or contamination is suspected.

The infant's diaper should be dry or, in the older child, sufficient time should have elapsed since the last voiding to insure the presence of urine in the bladder.  The child should be immobilized and the lower abdomen prepared as for blood culture. A syringe is fitted with a 22 gauge 1-1/2 inch needle.  The symphysis pubis is located and the needle inserted 1-2 cm above the symphysis <u>IN THE MIDLINE</u> at an angle 10-20° to the perpendicular aiming slightly caudad.  A perceptible change may be noted upon entering the bladder and with gentle suction the urine aspirated.

<u>NOTE</u>:  A digit in the rectum pushing anteriorly to compress the urethra prevents premature voiding and provides a measure of depth.

<u>Ref</u>:  Pediatrics <u>36</u>:132, 1965.

D.  TYMPANOPARACENTESIS

1. Patient is "mummified" in standard manner. Restraining belts placed across chest and knees. Head is held firmly by assistant.
2. <u>Anesthesia</u>:  Sedation is not usually necessary in infants and toddlers.  Sedation may be used with the larger child, more for the allaying of fear than for analgesia.  A cotton pledget saturated with a topical anesthetic gives good local anesthesia.
3. Cerumen is gently removed with a wire curette.
4. The tympanic membrane and canal are swabbed with tincture of zephiran.
5. A 2-1/2 ml plastic syringe containing approximately 1 ml sterile saline is attached to a No. 18 3-1/3 inch spinal needle that has a double bend to permit visualization of needle point.
6. Posterior inferior quadrant of tympanic membrane is visualized using an otoscope with operating head.
7. The tympanic membrane is perforated and maximum negative pressure is applied for a few seconds.
8. The first drop is smeared on an alcohol-cleaned slide for the gram stain.  One drop each on blood and chocolate agar plates and the rest into thioglycolate.

<u>NOTE</u>:  A culture of the canal after cleaning with Zephiran, but before puncturing, allows comparison with organisms obtained from aspirate.

E. PARACENTESIS

Valuable as a diagnostic or therapeutic test for
an abnormal collection of fluid within the peritoneal
cavity.

1. Precautions

If paracentesis is performed for therapeutic
measures, do not remove a large amount of fluid
too rapidly because hypovolemia and hypotension
may result from rapid fluid shifts.

2. Technique

Surgical preparation and draping of the abdomen
should be carried out.

a. With patient in supine position, needle aspiration is best carried out just lateral
to the rectus muscle in either the right or
left lower quadrants.
b. With patient in semi-Fowler or cardiac
position, a midline subumbilical aspiration
is desired.
c. Apply negative pressure as needle is inserted
into the peritoneal cavity.
d. Stop advancing needle once fluid appears in
the syringe. Continue aspiration slowly
with negative pressure until an adequate
amount of fluid has been obtained for diagnostic studies.
e. If upon entering the peritoneal cavity air
is aspirated, withdraw the needle immediately.
Aspirated air indicates entrance into a
hollow viscus. (In general, penetration of
a hollow viscus during paracentesis does not
lead to complications.) Paracentesis should
then be repeated with sterile equipment.

F. THORACENTESIS

Valuable as a diagnostic or therapeutic test for an
abnormal collection of fluid within the pleural
space.

Ideally, it should be performed with the patient
sitting on the side of the bed, with an assistant
standing in front to support him. Selection of the
interspace to be tapped is made on the basis of dull-
ness to percussion and the level of effusion on the
erect chest x-ray.

1.  Precautions

    Thoracentesis should be performed with care in
    order to avoid pneumothorax, lung puncture or
    trauma to vessels under the rib.

2.  Technique

    a.  Surgical preparation and draping of the
        chest should be carried out.
    b.  It is desirable to use a local anesthetic
        for the interspace to be entered.
    c.  A large bore needle attached to a 3-way
        stopcock and syringe are the necessary
        equipment. With needle bevel down, insert
        into pleural space on top of the rib.
    d.  As the pleural space is entered, negative
        pressure should be applied on the syringe.
    e.  The desired amount of fluid is then with-
        drawn slowly.
    f.  At the end of the procedure, the needle
        is withdrawn and a band-aid should be placed
        over the thoracentesis site.

    NOTE: One should get a follow-up chest x-ray after
    thoracentesis to rule out pneumothorax.

G. VENOUS CUTDOWN

    Readily accessible veins are the external jugular
    as it crosses the sternocleidomastoid muscle
    below the angle of the mandible, and the long
    saphenous just anterior to the medial malleolus.
    A venous cutdown should be performed under careful
    aseptic conditions and thereafter treated as a
    potential source of local and/or systemic infections.

    A surgical preparation of the skin is carried out
    and a transverse incision is made directly over the
    vein selected. The vein is isolated by blunt dis-
    section and two 3-0 silk sutures are placed about
    the vein. The distal ligature is then tied and used
    for traction. An oblique incision is made in the
    vein and the appropriate beveled silastic catheter,
    previously filled with saline, is inserted the
    desired length and the proximal ligature is tied
    snugly about the vein and catheter. The skin in-
    cision should be closed with fine silk and an addi-
    tional silk ligature about the catheter in the skin
    to secure the catheter externally. An antibiotic
    ointment is placed over the wound and a dressing is
    applied.

H.  VENOUS PRESSURE

1.  Equipment

    Syringe, saline, 3-way stopcock, spinal mano-
    meter and an 18-20 gauge needle (in smaller
    infants, a 22 or 23 gauge needle may be
    necessary).

2.  Technique

    a.  Assemble the 3-way stopcock with the syringe
        filled with sterile saline, the manometer
        placed vertically and the needle attached
        to the male hub.
    b.  Fill both the manometer and the needle with
        saline from the syringe.
    c.  With the infant supine, venipuncture a
        large vein.
    d.  Allow the saline from the manometer to run
        into the vein and read the pressure as the
        vertical distance in centimeters between
        the miniscus in the manometer and the right
        atrium.

3.  Precautions

    a.  Falsely elevated pressures:
        1)  Patient crying
        2)  Constriction of vein by an external
            pressure
        3)  Expiratory dyspnea
        4)  Positive pressure respirators
    b.  The larger the needle the more accurate
        the readings.
    c.  Manometer must be vertical.

4.  Use of Central Venous Cutdown

    If central venous cutdown is in superior vena
    cava for fluid administration, it may be used
    for venous pressure determinations if catheter
    is flushed before each reading.

5.  Normal Values

    Values depend very much on the position and size
    of the needle or catheter.  Average normal
    values differ and the individual's experience
    with the selected site and size of needle are
    important, but 8-12 cm $H_2O$ are generally
    accepted as normal.

I.  EXCHANGE TRANSFUSION

NOTE:  Hct, reticulocyte count, peripheral smear,
bilirubin, total protein, infant blood type and
Coomb's test should be performed on pre-exchange
sample of blood since they can no longer be of
diagnostic value on post-exchange blood.  If indicated, also save pre-exchange serum for serologic
studies.

1.  Routine Exchange:  for removal of sensitized
cells or bilirubin.

   a.  Cross match donor blood against maternal
       serum for first exchange and against post-
       change blood for subsequent exchanges.
   b.  Blood:
       1)  Type:  0 negative (low titer) anytime.
           Infant's type if no chance of maternal -
           infant incompatability.
       2)  Anticoagulant:  ACD or CPD unless
           infant is acidotic or hypocalcemic.
       3)  Temperature:  Room temperature.
       4)  Age:  fresh up to 48 hours old.
   c.  Infant feeding:  glucose-water p.o. or
       I.V. when exchange is indicated.  Empty
       stomach if infant was fed within 4 hours of
       exchange.
   d.  Albumin:  1 gram/kg I.V. 1-2 hours before
       exchange except before first exchange for
       hemolytic disease.
   e.  Procedure:
       1)  Provide for frequent monitoring and
           recording of heart and respiratory rates,
           temperature, color; a heat source;
           resuscitation equipment.
       2)  Prep and drape patient and operator for
           surgery.
       3)  Cut umbilical cord 1 cm or less from
           skin margin and find thin-walled vein.
       4)  Clear thrombi with forceps or catheter
           and insert catheter to:
           Minimum - until blood returns;
           Maximum - 1/2 to 2/3 of vertical
           distance from shoulder-tip to umbilicus.
           (see chart on page 286)
       5)  Measure venous pressure in cm of blood
           with ruler and record.  Repeat after
           each 100 ml exchanged.
       6)  Establish 20-30 ml deficit and use 20 ml
           increments in vigorous full-term infants.
           Smaller volumes for smaller, less stable
           infants.  Do not allow cells in donor
           unit to sediment.

7) Rate: 2-4 ml/kg/min avoiding mechanical trauma to patient and donor cells.
8) Calcium gluconate 10% solution: 1-2 ml slowly I.V. for tachycardia, irritability or prolonged Q-T segments. Rinse tubing with NaCl before and after. Observe for bradycardia during infusion.
9) Total volume exchanged should be 160 ml/kg up to one donor unit.
10) Use last withdrawal for: Hct, smear, bilirubin and future cross-matching.

2. Exchange for Anemic Heart Failure: Have O negative concentrated RBCs in the delivery room. Immediately measure the infant's venous pressure, establish a deficit and replace with enough RBCs to correct anemia and failure. Allow infant to stabilize for a few hours if possible before attempting a full two volume exchange.

3. Complications

a. Cardiovascular: Thrombo- or air emboli, thrombosis, arrhythmias, volume overload, cardiorespiratory arrest.
b. Chemical: Increased $K^+$, $Na^+$, decreased $Ca^{++}$, decreased glucose (esp. 2 hours post-exchange).
c. Hematological: Decreased platelets, over heparinization (may use 0.4 mg Protamine for each mg of heparin in donor unit).
d. Infectious: hepatitis, bacteremia.
e. Physical: injury to donor cells (especially from overheating), vascular or cardiac perforation, hypothermia.

H E M A T O L O G Y

A.  ROUTINE HEMATOLOGY
    (For normal values see Part IV-Reference Section)

1. <u>Hemoglobin Estimation</u>

Fill graduated tube of Sahli-Hellige Hemoglo-
binometer to the 10 mark with 0.1 N hydrochloric
acid (1 ml concentrated hydrochloric acid to
99 ml distilled water).  Obtain a drop of blood
and draw it into the pipette to the 20 cu mm
mark.  Wipe tip and blow contents into the
hydrochloric acid solution.  Rinse once.  Mix
with a mixing rod.  Let stand for 10 minutes.
Dilute the fluid with water drop by drop, mixing
after each addition, until it has exactly the
same color as the comparison standards.  The
graduation corresponding to the surface of the
fluid then indicates the percentage of hemoglobin.

2. <u>White Blood Cell Count</u>

Blood drawn up to the 0.5 mark and without delay
Turk's solution or 3% acetic acid drawn up to
11 mark.

Count number of cells in 4 large (1 mm) squares
after scanning with low power objective to
ascertain whether the cells are evenly distri-
buted.

Since each large square is 1 mm on the side,
and the coverslip lies 0.1 mm above the ruled
platform, the volume of each large square =
1 mm x 1 mm x 0.1 mm = 0.1 cu mm.

No. WBC/4 squares = No. WBC per 4 x 0.1 cu mm
                  = No. WBC per 0.4 cu mm
No. WBC in 1 cu mm = 10/4 x No. WBC in 0.4 cu
mm, since dilution is 0.5-11 or 1:20, No. WBC
per cu mm = No. WBC per 4 sq x 10/4 x 20 or
<u>No. WBC per 4 sq x 50.</u>

NOTE:  When the leukocyte count is low (below
4,000 cu mm) it is advisable for greater accuracy
to use 1:10 dilution.  When the WBC is very high,
it may be necessary to use the red cell counting
technique.

3. <u>Red Blood Cell Count</u>

Blood drawn up to the 0.5 mark, tip is wiped

clean and without delay diluting fluid (Hayem's solution or normal saline) is drawn up to the 101 mark.

Calculation: Area of 80 tiny squares = 80 x 0.0025 sq mm. R = No. of cells counted in 80 tiny squares, and blood has been diluted to 1:200. Then No. of cells in 1 cu mm = R x 200 x 1/0.02 = 10,000 R or <u>10,000 times the number of cells in 80 tiny squares</u>.

4.  <u>Eosinophil Count</u>

Blood is diluted 1:20 with a diluting fluid designed to cause lysis of red blood cells.

    2% aqueous eosin  0.5 ml
    Acetone           1.0 ml

Add distilled water to a total volume of 10 ml (can store in refrigerator for 2 weeks).

Using a hemoglobin pipette, draw blood to 0.02 ml and add 0.38 ml of diluting fluid (1/20 dilution). Both sides of a Fuchs-Rosenthal counting chamber are filled and counts made (chamber ruled to have 16 large squares each 1 x 1 mm, so total area is 16 sq mm. The depth is 0.2 mm; therefore, the volume of the ruled area is 3.2 cu mm).

If E = No. of eosinophils counted in one ruled area, then the absolute eosinophil count/cu mm of blood =

$$\frac{E \times 20}{3.2} = 6.25\ E$$

5.  <u>Platelet Count</u>

    a.  <u>Estimate</u>: An approximation of the platelet count on paired coverslips can be made from simple observation of the Wright's smear. If platelets are seen on the smear, severe thrombocytopenia can usually be ruled out. Always examine the periphery of the smear, as groups of platelets may be deposited in that area.

    NOTE: For rough approximation, 1 platelet/HPF corresponds to 10-15,000 platelets/mm$^3$.

    b.  Another estimate of the platelet count can

be made by looking at the ratio of RBC/
platelets per HPF. Normally this is approximately 20:1 (5 million/250,000).

Example: If 200 RBC's were present, there
should be 10 platelets present.
If only 5 were present with 200 RBC, the
approximate platelet count would then be
125,000/mm$^3$.

6. <u>Reticulocyte Count</u>

Add 5 drops of New methylene blue and 5 drops
of fresh, anticoagulated blood to a Wasserman
tube and mix. Allow to stand for 20 minutes.
Make a smear and mount on a slide. Count 500
red blood cells on two separate smears (total
1,000 RBCs). Number of reticulocytes reported
in percent.

7. <u>Wright's Staining Technique</u>

   a. Place the air-dried smear, film side up,
      on a staining rack.
   b. Cover smear with undiluted Wright's stain
      and leave for 1 minute.
   c. Dilute with distilled water (approximately
      equal volume) until a metallic scum appears.
      Allow this diluted stain to act for 2-1/2
      to 5 minutes.
   d. Without disturbing the slide, flood with
      distilled water and wash until thinner parts
      of film are pinkish red.

8. <u>Hematologic Indices</u>

   a. MEAN CORPUSCULAR HEMOGLOBIN (MCH)
      expresses ratio of hemoglobin to red cell
      count (the weight of hemoglobin in the
      average RBC) in absolute terms.

$$MCH = \frac{Hgb \ (gm\%) \ x \ 10}{RBC \ (millions \ per \ cu \ mm)}$$

      Result given in micromicrograms.

   b. MEAN CORPUSCULAR VOLUME (MCV) expresses the
      volume of the average RBC in absolute terms.

$$MCV = \frac{Hematocrit \ x \ 10}{RBC \ (millions \ per \ cu \ mm)}$$

      Result is given in cubic microns.

c. MEAN CORPUSCULAR HEMOGLOBIN CONCENTRATION
   (MCHC) measures in absolute terms the concentration of hemoglobin in the average RBC.

$$MCHC = \frac{Hgb \ (gm\%) \ x \ 100}{Hematocrit}$$

Result is expressed in per cent.

B. TESTS FOR BLEEDING TENDENCY

1. Bleeding Time (Ivy's Method)

   NOTE: Bleeding time should not be done using
   the ear lobe (Duke's method). Forearm safer.

   a. Place sphygmomanometer cuff around upper
      arm and inflate to 40 mm Hg.
   b. At a point below the fold at the antecubital
      fossa, and not overlying a vein, make
      incision 2 mm deep and 2 mm long. (Arm
      should hang down and blood should drop
      freely.)
   c. When first drop of blood appears, start
      timing. Blot drops with filter paper every
      30 seconds. Do not touch or manipulate
      wound.
   d. Record time when no further blood appears
      on paper. Normal: <6-1/2 minutes.

2. Clotting Time (Lee-White)

   a. Use 3 test tubes, 10 mm in diameter. Use
      size 18 or 20 needle. Rinse tubes, needle
      and syringe with sterile saline. Test
      tubes should be kept at body temperature by
      warming in hands or placing in incubator.
   b. Needle must enter vein on first attempt.
      Start timing.
   c. Remove needle and place 1 ml of blood in
      each tube, starting with tube #3. Do not
      squirt blood or shake tubes.
   d. Gently tilt tube #1 at 30 second intervals
      until it has clotted. Then tilt tube #2
      until clotting, and finally tilt #3.
      Record time tube #3 clots. This is clotting
      time.
   e. Normal: 6-12 minutes. (If siliconed tubes
      are used, time is approximately doubled.)

3. Clot Retraction

   Three ml of blood are put in a Wasserman tube.
   Incubate at 38°C. Inspect after 1 hour and

after 18-24 hours. Normally retraction of the
clot and expression of serum is appreciable
after 1 hour and marked after 18 hours. When
there is thrombocytopenia, polycythemia, or
very low fibrinogen levels, clot retraction is
delayed. Occasionally the clot of normal blood
fails to separate from the walls of the tube.
If the clot is loosened with an applicator,
however, retraction should occur promptly.

Because this test represents a summation of
the time required for both clotting and clot
retraction, it may be artificially prolonged in
the presence of a prolonged clotting time.

4. Clot Lysis

If fibrinogen levels are low (<50 mg%), a clot
will fall apart and resemble clot lysis.
Apparent lysis of a clot within 1 hour after
blood is drawn is abnormal. A normal person
should have continuation of a good clot at 24
hours.

5. Tourniquet Test (Rumpel-Leede)

a. Examine arm for petechiae and mark them.
b. Apply blood pressure cuff on upper arm
   and inflate midway between systolic and
   diastolic pressures.
c. Leave inflated cuff in place for 5 minutes.
d. Remove cuff, wait 5 minutes, and inspect
   arm, wrist and hand for petechiae.

If petechiae appear in large numbers earlier
than 5 minutes, release cuff immediately.

Comment:
a) Petechiae commonly appear in the antecubital area, volar aspect of the wrist.
b) Distribution of petechiae is usually
   irregular, and no effort should be made to
   count the number in a given area.
c) The test is graded 1+ to 4+, depending on
   whether there are a few or very many.
   Normally, only very occasional petechiae
   are found or none at all.

C. MISCELLANEOUS HEMATOLOGIC STUDIES

1. Sedimentation Rate (Wintrobe Method)

a. 5 ml venous blood is placed in oxalated
   or sequestrene bottle.

    b.  Place 1 ml of this in Wintrobe tube.
Determination should be done within 1 hour
after blood is obtained.

    c.  Place tube in special upright rack which
is balanced in vertical plane.

    d.  Read depth of fall of the red cell column
at the end of 60 minutes.

    e.  Normal values (mm/1 hr)

|  | Wintrobe | Westergren |
|---|---|---|
| Men | 0-8 | 1-3 |
| Women | 0-15 | 4-7 |
| Children | 4-20 | 0-2 |

    f.  Factors that increase rate of fall:
1) Anemia
2) Tilting
3) Warming

    g.  Factors or conditions with low or decreased
rate of fall:
1) Hypo- or afibrinogenemia
2) Old or cold blood
3) Excessive anticoagulant
4) Sickle cell anemia. Note: Oxygenate
sickle cell blood before performing ESR.
5) Congestive heart failure.
6) Polycythemia
7) Trichinosis

    h.  NOTE: "Correction" of sedimentation rate
for anemia is no longer recommended, but
simultaneous hematocrit should be recorded.

2. Sickle Preparation

Any substance which reduces oxygen tension will
cause the red cells of persons with sickle cell
anemia or trait to sickle.

    a.  Sulfite Solutions: A drop of 2% sodium
bisulfite or sodium hyposulfite may be used.
Capsules of sodium bisulfite are available
and the desired concentration is made fresh
every day. These preparations should be
read at 5 minutes, 60 minutes, 3 hours, and
12 hours.

    b.  BAL solution (fresh): Use 1 drop of 10%
injectable BAL plus 0.5 ml saline. Then
use 1 drop of the supernatant saline-BAL
mixture plus 1 drop of blood on coverslip.
Invert coverslip on slide and ring with
vaseline. Read at 5 minutes, 60 minutes,
3 hours, and 12 hours.

NOTE: Venous blood will sickle more readily
than capillary blood. A suggested method of
preparing the patient is to tourniquet the
finger with a rubber band for 5 minutes before
sticking the finger.

3. Osmotic Fragility (non-incubated) (Stanford's
   Method)

   a. To make 0.5% saline, add exactly 0.5 gm of
      pure, freshly dried sodium chloride to about
      50 ml of distilled water in 100 ml volu-
      metric flask, dissolve, and make up to
      volume with distilled water.
   b. Set up 2 rows of 12 small test tubes. One
      row is for the test on the patient's blood
      and the other for normal control.
   c. Number the tubes from left to right:
      25, 24, 23, 22, 21, 20, 19, 18, 17, 16,
      15, 14.
   d. With a capillary pipette, add to each tube
      the number of drops of 0.5% saline indicated
      by the number on the tube. With the same
      pipette, add the number of drops of distilled
      water needed to bring the contents of each
      tube to a total of 25 drops. Mix by shaking.
      The salt concentration in each tube is now
      the number on the tube multiplied by 0.02.
   e. Obtain blood by venipuncture and, with
      needle still attached to syringe, add one
      drop of blood to each tube. Mix.
   f. Let stand at room temperature for 2 hours.
      Record salt concentration at which there
      is first evidence of hemolysis (initial
      hemolysis). Record salt concentration at
      which no sediment of erythrocytes can be
      seen (complete hemolysis). Compare with
      control tubes.

      Normal range:
      1) Inital hemolysis (% Saline $\pm$ 1 S.D.)
         0.44 + 0.02
      2) Complete hemolysis (% Saline $\pm$ 1 S.D.)
         0.32 $\pm$ 0.02

NOTE: In some patients with congenital sphero-
cytic hemolytic anemia, the abnormality is not
detected unless osmotic fragility studies are
conducted on defibrinated blood which has been
incubated aseptically for 24 hours.

N E P H R O L O G Y

A.  ROUTINE URINALYSIS

1.  <u>Color</u>

    a.  <u>Endogenous</u>:
        1)  Yellow brown-deep brown:  bilirubin.
        2)  Red hues:  hemoglobin, RBC's, por-
           phyrins, urates.
        3)  Brown-black:  old blood, hemosiderin,
           myoglobin, homogentisic acid, melanin
           (especially if alkaline).
        4)  Purple-brown:  porphyrias (after
           specimen stands a few days).
        5)  Deep yellow:  riboflavin.
    b.  <u>Exogenous</u>:  See table on common exogenous
        urinary pigments on next page.

2.  <u>Clarity</u>

3.  <u>Specific Gravity</u>

    a.  Hydrometer.
    b.  Refractometer (American Optical Company
        T.S. Meter).  Requires only <u>1</u> drop of urine.
        Principle:  Refractive index of a solution
        is related to content of dissolved solids.

4.  <u>pH - Nitrazine Paper</u>

5.  <u>Albumin</u>

    a.  <u>Sulfosalicylic Acid Test</u>:
        1)  Add 8 drops of 20% sulfosalicylic acid
           to 1 ml of urine.
        2)  Mix equal amounts of urine and 3%
           sulfosalicylic acid.  This test can be
           quantitated with commercial standards.
        3)  False positives:  proteoses, tolbutamide,
           sulfonamides, penicillin, IVP dyes, PAS,
           phosphates, etc.
    b.  <u>Heat Test</u>:
        Heat urine until boiling.  If cloudiness
        occurs, add a few drops of 3% acetic acid.
        If cloudiness persists, it is due to albumin
        and not phosphate.
        Interpretation:  Faintly hazy $\pm$; definite
        haze 1+; cloud through which a print is
        legible 2+; heavier cloud 3+, immediate
        flocculation 4+.
    c.  <u>Albustix</u> (Ames Co.)

COMMON EXOGENOUS URINARY PIGMENTS

| Substances | Source | Color of Urine | |
|---|---|---|---|
| | | Acid | Alkaline |
| Anthracine Derivatives yielding chrysophanic acid (aloe, cascara, rhubarb, and senna) | Cathartics | Yellow-brown | Red-violet |
| Antipyrine | Analgesic | *Red | |
| Beets | Food | Red | Yellow |
| Bromsulphalein | Test dye | Colorless | Red |
| Congo Red | Test dye | Yellow | Red |
| Hedulin | Anticoagulant | Colorless | Red |
| Methylene Blue | Proprietary Drugs | Blue-Green | |
| Phenol | Poisoning | Colorless | Gradual oxidation of hydroquinone to olive to black pigment |
| Phenolphthalein | Cathartic | Colorless | Red |
| Phenolsulfonphthalein | Test dye | Colorless | Red |
| Povan | Antihelminthic | Red | |
| Pyridium | Analgesic | Red | Colorless |
| Red Candies | | Red | |
| Red Drug Flavorings | | Red | |
| Santonin | Antihelminthic | Yellow | Pink |
| Thymol | Antihelminthic | Colorless | Thymol hydroquinone turns olive on oxidation |

*pH changes not known

6. Reducing Substance

   a. Clinistix (Ames Co.): Specific for
      glucose; not for quantitation due to
      extreme sensitivity.
   b. Tes-tape (Eli Lilly Co.): Specific for
      glucose.
   c. Clinitest tablets (Ames Co.): Not speci-
      fic for glucose. 5 drops urine, 10
      drops water, 1 tablet. Compare with
      scale supplied. Reducing substances
      such as glucose, fructose, galactose,
      pentose (xylulose), lactose, ascorbic
      acid, chloramphenicol, and chloral
      hydrate all give positive tests with
      Clinitest. Sucrose does not react.

| | |
|---|---|
| Blue | Negative |
| Greenish blue | Trace |
| Green | 0.5% reducing substance |
| Greenish brown | 1% reducing substance |
| Yellow | 1.5% reducing substance |
| Brick red | 2% reducing substance |

7. Acetone

   a. Acetest tablets (Ames Co.)  ) Directions
   b. Acetone test power (Denver) )    from
   c. Ketostix (Ames Co.)        ) Manufacturer

8. Urine Gram Stain

   a. Purpose: To screen suspected urinary
      tract infections.
   b. Method: 1 drop of uncentrifuged clean
      catch or catheter obtained urine is
      Gram stained in usual manner.
   c. Interpretation: Almost all uncentri-
      fuged urine specimens with bacterial
      colony counts of $10^5$/ml or greater will
      have positive Gram stains. Obviously,
      a urine culture should be taken to
      confirm these results.

     Ref: Ped. 23:441, 1959.
          Ped. 26:441, 1960.

9. Sediment

Examine all fields for red cells, white
cells, casts and crystals. Area at edge of
coverslip should also be examined as formed
elements collect there. See illustration on
next page.

# URINARY SEDIMENTS

## Amorphous and Crystalline Chemical Sediments

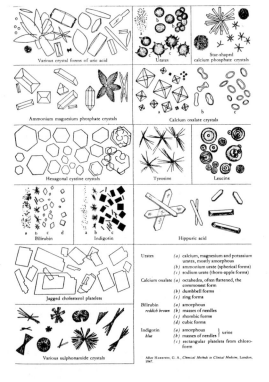

Various crystal forms of uric acid

Urates

Star-shaped calcium phosphate crystals

Ammonium magnesium phosphate crystals

Calcium oxalate crystals

Hexagonal cystine crystals

Tyrosine

Leucine

Bilirubin

Indigotin

Hippuric acid

Jagged cholesterol platelets

Various sulphonamide crystals

| Urates | (a) calcium, magnesium and potassium urates, mostly amorphous |
| | (b) ammonium urate (spherical forms) |
| | (c) sodium urate (thorn-apple forms) |
| Calcium oxalate | (a) octahedra, often flattened, the commonest form |
| | (b) dumbbell form |
| | (c) ring forms |
| Bilirubin reddish brown | (a) amorphous |
| | (b) masses of needles |
| | (c) rhombic forms |
| | (d) cubic forms |
| Indigotin blue | (a) amorphous |
| | (b) masses of needles |
| | (c) rectangular platelets from chloroform |

urine

After HARRISON, G. A., *Chemical Methods in Clinical Medicine*, London, 1947.

B.  MISCELLANEOUS URINALYSIS

    1.  <u>Tests for Urinary Reducing Substances Other Than Glucose</u>

        a.  <u>General</u>:  Qualitative Benedict's and Clinitest (Ames) tablets give similar results. Glucose oxidase strips Clinistix (Ames) and Tes-Tape (Lilly) are absolutely specific for glucose.  <u>Very rare</u> false negatives for glucose oxidase strips appear to be related to inhibition of enzyme in strip by compounds such as mercurials (e.g., Mercuhydrin).  It is not uncommon for <u>slight</u> discrepencies to exist between Clinitest and Clinistix results.

        b.  <u>Non-glucose Reducing Substances</u>:

| | |
|---|---|
| Ascorbic acid | Chloral hydrate |
| Fructose | Chloramphenicol |
| Galactose | Sulfonamides |
| Homogentisic acid | P.A.S. |
| Lactose | Tetracycline |
| Pentose (xylulose) | |
| Tyrosine and its derivatives in high concentration | |

           <u>Ref</u>:  BMJ <u>2</u>:745, 1968.

           <u>NOTE</u>:  Sucrose is <u>not</u> a reducing sugar.

        c.  <u>Specific Tests</u>
Sugar chromatography is most specific and can be performed by specialized labs.

    2.  <u>Cytomegalic Inclusion Disease</u>

        a.  <u>Purpose</u>:  Large epithelial cells with intranuclear inclusions are frequently found in the urine of patients, especially neonatal infants infected with human cytomegaloviruses.  Isolating the virus in culture and finding these cells in the body fluids is a practical antemortem method of making this diagnosis.  Absence of these cells in the urine does not exclude the diagnosis.

        b.  <u>Method</u>:
          1)  <u>Fresh</u> (!) urine is mixed 1:1 with 95% ethyl alcohol and centrifuged.
          2)  The sediment is placed on one slide and allowed to run onto serial slides resulting in thin smears that will air dry rapidly.
          3)  The smear is stained with toluidine

blue or hematoxylin and eosin.
4) Cells with intranuclear inclusions are
   sought under high dry magnification.
   The urine may also be passed through a
   milli-pore filter and the residue stained
   in situ and examined.

NOTE: The above methods can be applied to
a variety of body fluids.

Ref: Ped. 15:270, 1955.
     Am. J. Clin. Path. 22:424, 1952.

C. URINE TESTS FOR HEMOGLOBIN AND RELATED COMPOUNDS

1. Urine Hemoglobin

NOTE: A microscopic examination must be made to
differentiate hemoglobinuria from hematuria
(intact RBC's).

a. Occultest reagent tablets (Ames Co.):
   See directions on package.
b. Benzidine Test:
   1) Centrifuge urine and use sediment.
   2) Add 1 ml of saturated benzidine
      solution (in glacial acetic acid)
      and 1 ml of hydrogen peroxide.
   3) A bluish green color indicates hemoglobin.

c. Guaiac:
   1) Acidify 5 ml of urine with glacial
      acetic acid.
   2) Add guaiac solution drop by drop until
      cloudiness appears.
   3) Add hydrogen peroxide drop by drop.
   4) A blue color indicates hemoglobin.

A more specific test utilizes ether extraction.
To 10 ml urine add 1 ml glacial acetic acid and
10 ml ether. Shake thoroughly. Remove ether
layer to another tube and do guaiac test on
this material.

2. Urine Myoglobin

Dissolve 2.8 gm ammonium sulfate in 2 ml of
urine. Hemoglobin is precipitated, whereas
myoglobin stays in solution. Then repeat the
Benzidine test. Spectroscopic techniques are
more accurate.

3. <u>Urine Bilirubin</u>

    a. Icto Test (Ames Co.)
    b. Foam Test: Shake a few ml of urine.
       Yellow foam suggests bile.
    c. Bililabstix (Ames Co.).

4. <u>Urine Urobilinogen</u>

    a. Method:
       1) Remove bile from urine (see No. 5
          below.)
       2) Use 6-10 test tubes with the same
          diameter.
       3) Add 5 ml of water to all but the first
          tube.
       4) Add 5 ml urine to first and second tubes.
          Mix second tube and transfer 5 ml to
          third, etc.
       5) Add 0.5 ml Ehrlich aldehyde reagent
          <u>(Wallace and Diamond)</u>.
       6) Read last tube showing pink color.
          Must be read vertically with white paper
          under the test tube rack.

    b. Normal: 1:8-1:16 dilution.

    <u>Ehrlich Aldehyde Reagent</u>: 2 gm paradi-
    methylaminobenzaldehyde is dissolved in
    100 ml of 20% aqueous concentrated HCl.

5. <u>Urobilin (Schlesinger's Test)</u>

    If bilirubin is present, it must be removed.
    Add 2 ml 10% calcium chloride solution to 2 ml
    saturated sodium carbonate solution to 10 ml of
    urine. Filter or centrifuge, using filtrate or
    supernatant as below. A normal control should
    be run. For semi-quantitative purposes serial
    dilutions may be set up.

    To 10 ml of above filtrate (or to 10 ml of urine
    free of bile) add 1-2 drops of Lugol's solution.
    Add 10 ml of well-shaken Schlesinger's reagent.
    Filter and allow to stand for maximal develop
    ment of color. A green fluorescence indicates
    presence of urobilin; this is best seen when the
    test tube is viewed in bright sunlight against
    a black background or when light is concentrated
    upon it with a lens. Report test positive only
    when degree of fluorescence exceeds control.

      <u>Schlesinger's Reagent</u>
5 gm zinc acetate
95% alcohol qs ad 100 ml

<u>Lugol's Solution</u>
5 gm iodine
10 gm potassium iodide
Distilled water qs ad 100 ml

6. <u>Hemosiderin</u>

This may be seen as discrete golden granules in urinary sediment or may be present in casts. If such are seen, add a drop of 30% aqueous ammonium sulfite to a drop of urinary sediment. If the granules are hemosiderin, they will turn black (ferric sulfide).

A positive test indicates that hemoglobin has been passed into the renal tubules and there been converted to hemosiderin--usually the result of hemoglobinemia and hemoglobinuria. Hemosiderinuria may occur without manifest hemoglobinuria when the rate of excretion of hemoglobin is low. In paroxysmal nocturnal hemoglobinuria there is perpetual hemosiderinuria. It may also occur in hemochromatosis and intravascular hemolysis.

7. <u>Alternative Test for Hemosiderin</u>

a. Centrifuge 15 ml urine.
b. Mix sediment with 1 ml supernatant.
c. Add equal volume of 2 or 5% HCl.
d. To this mixture add 0.5 ml 10% aqueous solution of potassium ferrocyanide.

Positive test: Deep blue particles in sediment on microscopic examination.

D. RENAL FUNCTION TESTS

1. <u>Endogenous Creatinine Clearance</u>

a. <u>Purpose</u>: This is a good measure of glomerular filtration rate (GFR) and closely approximates the inulin clearance in the normal ranges of GFR. With the low GFR of advanced renal disease, it is above the inulin clearances.
b. <u>Method</u>: Timed collection of urine is made for any time period, recording the nearest minute. No poultry is fed. A single blood specimen is drawn during the collection

period unless the patient's renal function is rapidly changing. In the latter condition specimens are drawn at the beginning and end of the period. Hare and Hare method for true creatinine should be used.

c. Calculation:

$$Ccr = \frac{UV}{P} \times \frac{1.73}{S.A.}$$

NOTE: See pg. 260 for S.A. nomogram.

U   = urinary concentration of creatinine in mg%
V   = total volume of urine divided by number of minutes in the collection period = cc/min. (N.B. 24 hrs = 1440 mins.)
P   = serum creatinine level or average of 2 levels in mg%
S.A. = surface area in square meters (p. 260)

d. Normal Values:
1) Newborns and Prematures:
40-65 ml/min/1.73 sq meters
2) 1-1/2 Years and Older:
a) Males
124 + 25.8 ml/min/1.73 sq meters
b) Females
108.8 + 13.5 ml/min/1.73 sq meters
3) Adults:
a) Males
105 + 13.9 ml/min/1.73 sq meters
b) Females
95.4 + 18 ml/min/1.73 sq meters

Ref: New Eng. J. Med. 266:317, 1962.
Acta Paed. 48:443, 1959.

2. Dilution and Concentration Test

a. Concentration
A random urine S.G. of 1.023 or more indicates intact concentrating ability within the limits of clinical testing and no further tests are indicated.

Technique: After a dry evening meal fluids are withheld for 12 hours. Normally, the urine S.G. will reach 1.023 or more under these conditions. If, at 12 hours concentration, this is not evident, pitressin responsiveness may be determined. (5 units vasopressin IM with sp.gr $\geq$ 1.023 2-8 hours after injection)

Caution: Fluid deprivation for only a few
hours in the face of impaired concentrating
ability can lead to dehydration, hypernatremia,
and hypovolemic shock. Serial observations
of body weight, hematocrit, serum protein,
and serum sodium or osmolality are essential. Do not progress if patient loses 8%
of body weight.

Ref: AJDC 114:639, 1967.

b. Dilution
Normally, if the fluid intake is increased
to cause maximum diuresis, the S.G. will
fall to 1.003 or less. Dilution tests are
dangerous in patients with reduced GFR and
rarely used.

Technique: 20-30 ml/kg of water (maximum
1000 ml) is ingested over 30-45 minutes.
Voided specimens checked over the next 3
hours should reveal a S.G. of 1.003 or
below. This is not a standard water load
test.

3. Three Glass Test

With a full bladder initially, the patient is
asked to void 2-3 ounces into a glass. This
specimen will contain washings from the urethra.
A similar amount is passed into a second glass;
a sample of bladder urine. The prostate is then
massaged and a third glass obtained supposedly
containing bladder and prostatic secretions.
Examine each specimen for formed elements and
culture each.

4. Addis Count

a. Purpose: Allows quantitation and standardi-
zation of the excretion of formed elements
in the urine and is relatively free of error
due to change in urine flow rate. Test is
pointless if routine microscopic examination
of the urine is positive.

b. Method: Fluid is restricted after 8 a.m.
for adults or after 4 p.m. for children.
Urine is collected from 7 p.m. to 7 a.m.
Collection started after a voiding and timed
accurately. Add 0.5 ml 40% formalin to
collection bottle. Urine must be acid.

The amount of urine excreted in 1/5 hour is
placed in a graduated centrifuge tube and
spun for 5 minutes at 1800 rpm. All but
0.5 ml of supernatant is removed with pipette.
The sediment is resuspended and dropped
onto a counting chamber. The coverslip
is set down on the drop, not slid into
place. The number of elements in a large
square (0.1 mm$^3$) x 100,000 equals the
daily output.

c.  Normal:

|        | Children      | Newborns, 0-6 days |
|--------|---------------|--------------------|
| RBC    | 1,000,000/d   | 6,000,000/d        |
| WBC    | 2,000,000/d   | 13,000,000/d       |
| Casts  | 10,000/d      | 400,000/d          |

Ref:  Acta Paed. 50:361, 1961.

5.  Orthostatic Albuminuria

a.  Purpose: This is a fairly common type of
proteinuria usually seen in the absence of
significant renal disease. Since patients
with true renal disease may show the same
phenomenon, the diagnosis must be made by
exclusion if there is (1) no impairment
of renal function, (2) no hypertension,
(3) no urinary abnormality other than
proteinuria or an increased number of casts,
at least 90% hyaline.

b.  Method:
1)  No fluids after 6 p.m.
2)  Empty bladder immediately before
    retiring and discard this urine.
3)  Remain flat in bed during night. Any
    urine voided during night is discarded.
4)  Collect a voided specimen immediately
    after waking in bed in the morning.
    Label #1
5)  Drink 2 glasses of water. Stand erect
    and quietly for 20 minutes, then void
    and label #2.
6)  Kneel on a chair for 20 minutes with
    the back arched backward as much as
    possible. Then void and label #3.
7)  Walk about actively for 30 minutes, then
    void and label #4.

For each specimen record the specific gravity
and the protein content, by the heat and
acetic acid, sulfosalicylic or other simple
test.

In orthostatic albuminuria urine excreted in recumbent position contains no albumin. Urine excreted in upright or lordotic positions contains variable amounts of albumin.

6. Urine Acidification Test

   a. Purpose: In order to evaluate the renal tubular acidification mechanisms when random urine pH values are greater than 6 in the presence of systemic metabolic acidosis a challange with ammonium chloride may be required.

   b. Method:
      1) Ammonium chloride 5.5 mEq/kg (150 mEq/m2) is given orally.
      2) Over the next 5 hours urine pH should be measured every hour if possible.
      3) Plasma bicarbonate concentration should be measured 3 hours after ingestion of ammonium chloride.

   c. Results: The urine pH should fall below 5.5. If urine pH is not lower than 5.5 and the plasma bicarbonate is not below 17 mEq/L, larger doses of ammonium chloride may be necessary to produce a plasma bicarbonate concentration below an abnormal renal bicarbonate reabsorption threshold. Extreme care should be taken when using larger doses of ammonium chloride.

   d. Interpretation:

   Normal Response
   1) Fall in plasma bicarbonate concentration.
   2) Fall in urine pH to below 5.5.

   Renal Tubular Acidosis - Distal (Type I)
   Males=Females
   1) Fall in plasma bicarbonate concentration.
   2) Urine pH remains above 6.0.

   Renal Tubular Acidosis - Proximal (Type II)
   Male>>Females
   1) Fall in plasma bicarbonate concentration (see above).
   2) Fall in urine pH below 5.5.

   NOTE: Urine pH of 5 does not R/O the diagnosis of a proximal RTA and a simultaneous plasma bicarbonate is essential.

   Ref: Ped. Res., 1:452, 1967.

# C E R E B R O S P I N A L   F L U I D

<u>CAUTION</u>:  Lumbar puncture may be dangerous in the pre-
sence of increased intracranial pressure and overlying
skin infections, as well as in individuals who have
bleeding tendencies.

Prior to lumbar puncture funduscopic examination should
be done.  Presence of papilledema calls for extreme
caution and may contraindicate lumbar puncture.

Sudden drop in pressure by rapid release of spinal
fluid may be fatal in presence of increased pressure.

In those patients with thrombocytopenia, a platelet count
above $50,000/mm^3$ is desirable prior to LP.

1.  <u>Cerebrospinal Fluid Pressure</u>
    The patient should lie quietly on his side with head
    and lower extremities only gently flexed.  Compression
    of the abdomen should be avoided.  If these qualifi-
    cations are not met, the spinal fluid pressure may be
    artifically elevated.  The manometer should be
    attached to the needle with care to prevent the loss
    of fluid, for this will lower the pressure.  There
    should be free flow of fluid, and usually fluctuations
    are noted with respirations.  Several readings should
    be made and recorded as mm. of cerebrospinal fluid.

    <u>Queckenstedt Test</u>:
    (SHOULD NOT BE DONE IN PRESENCE OF INCREASED
    INTRACRANIAL PRESSURE.)  Compress first the right
    and then the left jugular veins.  Normally this will
    produce a rise in intracranial pressure which in turn
    will be transmitted to the lumbar canal.  Failure of
    spinal fluid pressure to rise indicates either ob-
    struction in the lumbar canal or obstruction in the
    ipsilateral venous system (acquired or congenital).

2.  <u>Collection of Cerebrospinal Fluid</u>
    Collect 3 tubes of spinal fluid under sterile pre-
    cautions (save a fourth tube if possible for addi-
    tional studies).  The first tube is for culture, the
    second for chemistry determinations and the third for
    cell count.  About 1-2 ml in each tube will suffice
    for routine examinations, but cell count and gram
    stain can be done on less than 1 ml.  Larger amounts
    of fluid should be collected if special studies are
    contemplated (i.e., guinea pig innoculation, col-
    loidal gold, etc.).

3.  <u>Pandy Test</u>

    A qualitative test for increased spinal fluid

protein. It begins to become positive at CSF protein
levels of about 50 mg%.

A drop of spinal fluid is allowed to fall into 2 ml
of saturated (5%) phenol solution (Pandy solution).
DO NOT SHAKE. If protein is increased, a cloud will
form. This is recorded 1 to 4+ depending on the
degree of cloudiness. Pandy solution and spinal
fluid should be at the same temperature; otherwise,
a false positive test may be obtained.

4. Appearance

   Record:
   a. Color
   b. Clarity
   c. Presence or absence of pellicle

5. Culture

   Spinal fluid culture should be planted as soon as
   possible. Follow instructions in MICROBIOLOGICAL
   EXAMINATIONS using sterile precautions. Drop CSF
   directly onto appropriate media and also incubate
   remaining CSF as original fluid. Time may be saved
   by placing sensitivity discs on a second set of
   streaked plates.

6. Cell Count

   Unacidified spinal fluid is examined microscopically
   in the counting chamber. The presence of RBC's and
   crenation are noted. RBC's should be counted. Then
   rinse pipette with glacial acetic acid, and allow to
   stand for 5 minutes. Then count WBC's on all 9
   chambers and multiply by 10/9. The pipette may be
   rinsed with a stain to hemolyze the red cells and
   accentuate the white cells.

   Do not attempt a differential WBC count on the
   cells in the counting chamber. These counts are
   inaccurate.

7. Differential WBC and Cell Morphology

   a. A drop of centrifuged CSF is placed on a slide
      and caused to run down its length. This forms
      a thin smear which dries quickly before cell
      forms are distorted. It can be stained with
      Wright's stain.
   b. If leukemic meningitis is suspected, or cell
      morphology is critical, fresh CSF is added to
      the patient's serum in equal parts immediately,
      and a stained smear made.

8. Examination for Bacteria

   a. If pellicle forms, it should be fished out,
      crushed between 2 clean slides and the slides
      pulled apart, giving 2 smears. One is stained
      with Gram's stain and the other for acid-fast
      bacillus.
   b. Uncontaminated CSF is spun, and the sediment is
      smeared on a slide and Gram stained.
   c. If the Gram stain reveals suspected H. flu or
      pneumococci, a Quellung may be set up.

9. Examination for Fungus

   One drop of CSF and 1 drop of either Nigrosin or
   dilute India Ink are placed on a slide and mixed
   well. Cover with coverslip and press out excess
   fluid. Ring with vaseline. Examine for round
   organisms with large halos. If your index of suspi-
   cion for fungi is high you may incubate the preparation at $37^\circ$ and reexamine at 24 and 48 hours.

10. Chemical Determinations

   a. Sugar:
      1) Send stat to chemistry lab, or
      2) Freeze for glucose oxidase determination,
         or
      3) Add 0.1 ml of spinal fluid to 1.9 ml
         phosphotungstic acid and send to chemistry
         lab at later time.

      Rapid semi-quantitative: Place 1.0 ml Benedict's
      solution in each of 6 Wassermann tubes. Add
      0.05, 0.1, 0.15, 0.20, and 0.25 ml of spinal
      fluid. Tube #6 is a control. Place in boiling
      water bath for 5 minutes. Reduction (green
      color) should occur in 2 or 3 tubes.

   b. Protein: Send to chemistry laboratory.

11. Serologic Studies

   May be performed in serology laboratory.

## S Y N O V I A L   F L U I D

A. EXAMINATION OF SYNOVIAL FLUID

1. Appearance

   Note quantity, turbidity, pH, clot formation, viscosity, and icterus.

2. Microscopic

   Examine undiluted for total RBC and WBC count and crystals. Dilute with saline to obtain WBC if necessary. The use of acid WBC diluting fluids may produce clotting.

   Normal cell count: less than 180 WBC/mm$^3$, with less than 25% polys.

3. Chemical

   Obtain sugar and protein determinations. Sugar should be within 10 mg% of blood sugar. Be sure to obtain simultaneous blood sugar.

4. Mucin

   To 1 ml synovial fluid from which the cells have been centrifuged, add 4 ml water, then 2-3 drops glacial acetic acid, and stir. A tight rope of mucin is normal. In infection and rheumatoid arthritis no precipitate or a loose fibrillar precipitate is formed.

5. Bacteriologic

   Gram stain sediment, and culture aerobically, anaerobically, and for AFB.

6. Icterus

   May indicate trauma. Sample sent to chemistry lab for bilirubin.

NOTE: A portion of the fluid may be placed in a heparinized tube to prevent clotting.

B. CHARACTERISTICS OF SYNOVIAL FLUIDS IN DISEASE

| Etiology | Appearance | Leukocytes/mm³ (mean#) | % Neutrophils (mean %) | Mucin | *Glucose (mean) Difference mg/100 ml |
|---|---|---|---|---|---|
| Normal | Clear, straw | 13-200 (63) | 0-25 (6.5) | Good, tight | 10 or less |
| Traumatic | Clear, straw or hemorrhagic | 200-5800 (1680) | 0-36 (10) | Good, tight | 10 or less |
| Degenerative | Clear, yellow | 70-1950 (520) | 0-58 (8) | Good, tight | 10 or less |
| Rheumatic Fever | slightly turbid, yellow | 1,000-63,000 (10,000) | 8-98 (46) | Good, tight | 10 or less |
| Gout | Turbid | 1,000-31,000 (10,000) | 48-94 (83) | Loose, friable | 0-40 |
| Rheumatoid | Clear to turbid, yellow-green | 600-66,000 (15,000) | 5-96 (65) | Loose, friable | 0-30 |
| Tuberculosis | Turbid, yellow | 2,500-105,000 (25,000) | 29-96 (67) | Loose, friable | 0-108 (57) |
| Gonorrheal | Turbid, yellow | 1,500-108,000 (15,000) | 2-96 (65) | Loose, friable | 0-97 (26) |
| Septic | Very turbid | 25,000-200,000 (65,000) | 75-100 (95) | Loose, friable | 50-120 (70) |

*Refers to difference between glucose concentration in joint fluid and fasting blood sugar.

M I C R O B I O L O G I C A L

E X A M I N A T I O N S

A.  EXAMINATION OF FRESH PREPARATIONS AND STAINED
    SMEARS

    NOTE:  Thin smears are best for staining.  When
    "fixing" smears do not overheat; several passes
    through a flame are sufficient.  Cool slide in air
    before staining.

    1.  Staining Techniques

        a.  Gram Stain (Rapid Method):
            1)  Flood slide with gentian violet --
                15 seconds.
            2)  Wash, add Gram's iodine -- leave 20
                seconds, decolorize with acetone
                alcohol -- 5 seconds.
            3)  Wash with water.
            4)  Counterstain with safranin -- 15 seconds.

        b.  Acid Fast Stain:
            1)  Flood slide with Kenyoun's stain --
                5 minutes.  Wash with water.
            2)  Decolorize with acid alcohol until
                faint pink.  Wash with water.
            3)  Counterstain with 1/2% methylene blue --
                1 minute.

        c.  India Ink (Nigrosin's Stain):
            A negative stain used mainly for identification
            of Cryptococcus.  India Ink must be quite dilute.
            One drop of test fluid and one drop of India Ink
            are mixed well and examined for presence of
            organism identified as a refractile image against
            a black background.  (see technique under CSF
            examination for fungus pg.33)

B.  CULTURE METHODS

    1.  The Following Material Should Be Cultured
        Immediately:

        a.  Blood:
            1)  Approximately 2 ml blood into thiogly-
                colate media.
            2)  Approximately 8 ml blood into screw-
                capped bottle of infusion broth.

            NOTE:  If patient is being treated with
            penicillin, use 0.2 + 0.5 ml of penicilli-
            nase respectively in each.  Also culture the

the penicillinase in thioglycolate as a
control for contamination.

    b.  CSF:
       1)  Chocolate agar (place in $CO_2$ jar).
       2)  Human blood agar.
       3)  Desoxycholate agar.
       4)  Thioglycolate.
       5)  Original fluid.

    c.  Urine:
       1)  One loopful (special loop) per plate.
       2)  Human blood agar.
       3)  Desoxycholate agar plate.
       4)  Incubate.

    d.  Cavity Fluids:
       1)  Culture the same as CSF fluid.
       2)  Peritoneal and abscess cultures
          should be taken directly to lab for
          special anaerobic cultures.

2.  All Other Specimens:

Throat, Ear, NP, Eye, Skin (wound abscess),
Stool (rectal swabs):  Place swab in transfer
media and refrigerate.

3.  To expedite cultures (evenings and weekends)
the house officer may use the following:

    a.  NP, Eye and Ear:
       1)  Human blood agar.
       2)  Desoxycholate agar.
       3)  Chocolate blood agar.
       4)  Swab in transport media.

    b.  Throat:
       1)  Human blood agar.
       2)  Desoxycholate agar.
       3)  Swab in transport media.

    c.  Vagina and Urethra:
       1)  Thayer-Martin agar
       2)  Human blood agar.
       3)  Chocolate blood agar.
       4)  Thioglycolate broth.
       NOTE:  Always culture immediately and always
       do gram stain as well.

    d.  Skin:
       1)  Human blood agar.
       2)  Desoxycholate agar.
       3)  Inoculate thioglycolate.

NOTE: The house officer may elect to place sensitivity discs on the plates of cultures from those patients in whom a rapid answer is critical.

4. Fungus Preparation

Edges of a lesion in which fungus is suspected may be scraped with a scalpel onto a glass slide. The scrapings are covered with 10% to 20% KOH or NaOH and a coverslip applied. Warm over light globe for a few minutes. Examine for fragments of mycelia and spores.

## S T O O L   E X A M I N A T I O N

1.  Parasitology Preparations - See next page for illus-
    trations.

    a.  Direct Smear:  Add small amount of feces to
        drop of saline, mix and remove feces with
        applicator stick.  Cover.  Examine under low
        power to locate the parasite and high dry for
        identification.  Species identification of
        protozoan cysts can be made by adding iodine
        stain (KI 1.0% saturated with crystalline
        iodine) to smear, or by making an additional prep
        in a drop of stain.

2.  Examination for Pinworms

    a.  Parents inspect perianal area at night about
        an hour after the child retires, looking for
        thread-like white worms (1/4 to 1/2 inch).
    b.  Pinworm Smear:  Cellophane Tape Method
        1)  Obtain smear in morning before bath.
        2)  Cover one end of a tongue depressor with
            cellophane tape, sticky side out.
        3)  Apply to perianal area with mild pressure.
        4)  Put 1 drop xylol on glass, then apply
            tape to slide.
        5)  Look for ova under microscope.
    c.  Examination of Stool after Purgative and Enema.

3.  Test for Occult Blood in Stool (Guaiac Method)

    Reagents:
        Gum guaiac
        Glacial acetic acid
        Hydrogen peroxide (fresh)

    a.  Method #1:  Make thin smear of stool on filter
        paper.  Serially apply 2 drops of each in this
        order:  acetic acid, guaiac, hydrogen peroxide.
        A royal blue color is 4+; a green color is
        negative.  Other gradations of blue are 1-3+.
        1)  Medicinal iron does not give a positive
            guaiac reaction.
    b.  Method #2:  Pour an equal amount of this reagent
        over the stool dilution.  A blue color will
        form if positive.  Several minutes should be
        allowed.

4.  Apt Test for Fetal Hemoglobin

    a.  Method:  Mix specimen (stool, vomitus, etc.)
        with an equal quantity of tap water.  Centri-
        fuge or filter.  Supernatant must have pink
        color to proceed.  To 5 parts of supernatant,
        add 1 part of 0.25 N (1%) NaOH.

# DIFFERENTIAL CHARACTERISTICS OF
# IMPORTANT HUMAN ROUNDWORM OVA

## Ascaris lumbricoides

Infertile Egg                          Fertile Eggs

Surface View          Optical Section

| Trichuris trichiura | Red Blood Cells at same Magnification as ova ... for size comparison | Enterobius vermicularis |
|---|---|---|
|  |  |  |

Stages of Development of Necator americanus or
Ancylostoma doudenale

| Strongyloides stercoralis | PROTOZOA | |
|---|---|---|
| | Giardia | Entamoeba histolytica |
|  |  |  |
| | Cyst | Trophozoite |

*Margaret Showers 1972*

b. Interpretation: A pink color persisting over 2 minutes indicates fetal hemoglobin. Adult hemoglobin gives a pink color that becomes yellow in 2 minutes or less.

Ref: J. Pediat. 47:6, 1955.

5. TCA Test for Protein in Meconium

a. Method: Mix meconium with 2 to 8 ml of water. Allow to stand at room temperature for 1 hour and then centrifuge. Filter supernatant. Mix 0.25 ml of filtered supernatant with 0.25 ml of 20% trichloroacetic acid.
b. Interpretation: If original meconium contains protein a voluminous precipitate is formed. In patients with meconium ileus this strongly suggests pancreatic insufficiency.

Ref: Peds, 21:635, 1958.

6. Farber Meconium Test

a. Purpose: Helpful in diagnosing intestinal atresia of newborn.
b. Method: Thin smear of meconium is made using central portion of the specimen to avoid contamination by epithelial cells from the anal area. Place slide in ether for 5 minutes and then allow to dry. Stain for 1 minute with Sterling's gentian violet (5 gm gentian violet, 10 ml 95% alcohol, 2 ml aniline dye, 88 ml water). Wash slide in $H_2O$, decolorize with acid alcohol and dry.
c. Interpretation: In cases of intestinal atresia the contents of the amniotic sac are absent from meconium. Normally, cornified epithelial cells (large thin scales without nuclei) are abundant in meconium.

7. Stool Gelatinase (Trypsin) Activity

a. Purpose: Infants and young children (less than 4 years) normally have measurable gelatinase activity in their stools. This is mostly contributed by the pancreas although small and usually insignificant amounts are added by some bacteria. Low amounts found in constipation, marasmus, pancreatic insufficiency and pancreatic duct obstruction.

b. Method:
1) To 4 ml of water, add enough stool to bring the total volume to 5 ml (1:5 dilution). Mix well and centrifuge. Run a control stool in a similar way.
2) Make 1:10 dilution by adding 1 ml of supernatant from above to 1 ml of water. Make 1:50, 1:100, 1:200 dilutions in a similar way.
3) Cut undeveloped x-ray film into long narrow strips and insert each into long test tubes containing the dilutions.
4) Incubate at 37°C for 1 hour.
5) Record the highest dilution that digests the gelatin from the film.

c. Interpretation: The normal child has a titer of 1:100 or greater. A control stool should always be run. Some children with partial pancreatic insufficiency may have occasional stools with normal amounts due to maximal stimulation of remaining pancreatic tissue from the ingestion of food. Therefore, low titers are more significant than high ones.

8. <u>Microscopic Stool Fat Test</u>

A drop of stool and 2 drops of 1% scarlet red in absolute alcohol (or Sudan IV) are mixed on a slide and mixed with 1 drop of saline. A coverslip is placed over the slide. The fat present may appear as round droplets stained red, or as clumps of spindle-shaped crystals stained faint orange or not stained at all. An excessive number of fat droplets or crystals is characteristic of any form of steatorrhea.

<u>Ref</u>: Am. J. Dis. Child. <u>69</u>:141, 1945.

9. <u>Microscopic Stool Starch Test</u>

A drop of stool not more than a few hours old is mixed on a slide with 1 drop of normal ammonium chloride, and then with 1 drop of 3.5% solution of iodine in 5% potassium iodide. Starch granules stain blue, but the free granules must be distinguished from those enclosed in vegetable cells. Normally, free extracellular granules are not frequent but with defects in starch digestion such guanules may be present in large numbers. Intracellular starch granules may be ignored except when they occur in very great numbers.

10. Test for Sugar in Stool

    a.    Purpose:  Detection of carbohydrate malabsorption by measuring reducing substances in stool. Since sucrose is not a reducing substance modify test as noted.

    b.    Method:
        1)  Place a small amount of fresh liquid stool in a test tube.
        2)  Dilute with twice its volume of water. For sucrose use 1N HCl instead of water and boil briefly.
        3)  Place 15 drops of this suspension in 2nd test tube containing a Clinitest tablet.
        4)  Compare the resulting color with the chart provided for urine testing.

    c.    Interpretation:  Normally one finds 0.25% or less reducing substances in the stool. Values of 0.25% to 0.5% are questionable. The finding of 0.5% or greater reducing substances in the stool is abnormal and suggests carbohydrate malabsorption.

M E T A B O L I C   T E S T S

A.  TOLERANCE TESTS

    1.  Oral Glucose Tolerance Test
        a.  Purpose:  To test both absorption and
           metabolism of glucose.
        b.  Patient preparation:  Must ingest adequate
           diet for 3 days and be NPO for 12 hours
           preceding start of test.
           Adequate diet: 50% of total calories
           as carbohydrate
           Total calories:
           0-12 months - minimum of 100 calories
             kg/day
           1-12 years - 1000 calories + 100 calories
             for every year of age
        c.  Dosage:
           1.75 grams/kg body weight with a maximum
            dose of 100 grams

           Mix glucose with water and lemon juice
           as a 20 per cent solution.  If not taken
           well, gavage.

        d.  Specimens: Capillary or venous blood.
           Source should be consistent throughout a
           single test.
        e.  Time:  0 minutes, 1/2 hour, 1 hour, 2
           hours, 3 hours.  (Add 4 and 5 hour
           specimens when evaluating hypoglycemia.)
        f.  Urine:  Collect at 0, 1 and 2 hours and
           analyze for sugar.
        g.  Interpretation:  Peak blood glucose at 1/2-
           1 hour.  Usually at or near fasting level
           at 2 hours.  Glucose quantitation varies
           depending on whether assayed by true glucose
           (glucose oxidase) or reducing substance
           method and source of blood sample.

| Normal Values When Total Reducing Substance Measured Using Capillary Blood | | | | | | |
|---|---|---|---|---|---|---|
| Time: 0 | 1/2 hr | 1 hr | 2 hr | 3 hr | 4 hr | 5 hr |
| Mg%: 101±3 | 162±9 | 131±7 | 108±6 | 91±5 | 91±3 | 94±3 |

The above values are based on capillary blood which was
quickly lysed with distilled water and precipitated
with tungstic acid.

United States Public Health Service Criteria For Interpretation of Oral Glucose Tolerance Test Results (determination of true glucose on capillary whole blood):

| | | |
|---|---|---|
| Fasting | >110 milligram % | = 1 point |
| 1 hour | >170 milligram % | = 1/2 point |
| 2 hours | >120 milligram % | = 1/2 point |
| 3 hours | >110 milligram % | = 1 point |

A total of 2 points is diagnostic of diabetes. A sum of 1 or 1 1/2 points is considered suspect and is an indication for repeating.

2. <u>IV Glucose Tolerance Test</u>

   a. <u>Purpose</u>: Obviates problems of absorption found in oral test.
   b. <u>Method</u>: Glucose 0.5 gm/kg in a 20-50% solution is given over 2 to 4 minutes.
   c. <u>Specimens</u>: Determine blood glucose at 0, 5, 15, 30, 45, and 60 minutes.
   d. <u>Urine</u>: Collect before and at end of test.
   e. <u>Normal</u>: Peak value comes at 5 minutes and normal should be attained at 45-60 minutes.

3. <u>Glucagon Tolerance Test</u>

   a. <u>Purpose</u>: Glucagon increases blood sugar by stimulating liver glycogenolysis and gluconeogenesis.
   b. <u>Method</u>: Patient NPO 4-12 hours as tolerated. Glucagon 30 micrograms/kg (maximum 1 milligram) given IV.
   c. <u>Specimens</u>: Measure blood glucose at 0, 10, 20, 30, 40, 60, and 90 minutes.
   d. <u>Normal</u>: Blood glucose rises 40-60% in 30 minutes. Diminished to absent response in glycogen storage disease types I, III, VI, VIII, IX, X and severe hepatocellular disease.

   <u>Ref</u>: J. Ped. <u>82</u>: 558, 1973.

4. <u>Oral Galactose Tolerance Test</u>

   a. <u>Purpose</u>: The conversion of galactose to glucose requires hepatic glucose-6-phosphatase activity which is deficient in type I glycogen storage disease. <u>THIS TEST SHOULD NOT BE USED IN GALACTOSEMIA OR GALACTOKINASE DEFICIENCY</u>.

b. <u>Method</u>: Patient NPO 4-12 hours as tolerated. Galactose 3 gm/kg is administered
orally as a 20% solution over 3 minutes.
c. <u>Specimen</u>: Determine blood glucose and
lactate at 0, 15, 30, 45, and 60 minutes.
d. <u>Normal</u>: See IV galactose test.

5. <u>IV Galactose Tolerance Test</u>

a. <u>Purpose</u>: Same as oral galactose test. This
test may be safer in glycogen storage
disease type I because of lower galactose
load.
b. <u>Method</u>: Patient NPO 4-12 hours as tolerated. Galactose 1 gm/kg as a 20% solution
IV over 3 minutes.
c. <u>Specimen</u>: Determine blood glucose and
lactate at 0, 10, 20, 30, 45 and 60 minutes.
d. <u>Normal</u>: Significant elevation in blood
glucose without a change in blood lactate.
In type I glycogen storage disease blood
glucose does not change while blood lactate
increases 2-4 fold. <u>May precipitate
symptomatic lactic acidosis</u>.

Ref: Pediat. <u>19</u>:585, 1957.

6. <u>Fructose Tolerance Test</u>

a. <u>Purpose</u>: The normal conversion of fructose
to glucose is blocked in both hereditary
fructose intolerance and type I glycogen
storage disease. In hereditary fructose
intolerance (fructose-1-phosphate aldolase
deficiency) this test results in nausea,
vomiting, hypoglycemia, hypophosphatemia,
hypokalemia and fructosuria.
b. <u>Method</u>: Fructose 0.25 gm/kg in adult or
3 gm/M$^2$ in children by rapid IV injection.
Dose may be increased if result equivocal.
c. <u>Specimens</u>: Measure blood glucose, and
phosphate at 0, 10, 20, 30, 45 and 60
minutes. Check Dextrostix on each sample.
d. <u>Interpretation</u>: Normally a significant
elevation in blood glucose occurs. In
hereditary fructose intolerance serum
inorganic phosphate falls first, followed by a
prolonged decrease in blood sugar. <u>50%
GLUCOSE SOLUTION SHOULD BE AT BEDSIDE</u>.
(Dose 1-2 ml/kg)

Ref: E. Froesch in <u>The Metabolic Basis
of Inherited Disease</u>; (Stanbury,
Wyngaarden and Fredrickson, eds),
McGraw Hill, 1972.

7. Tolbutamide Tolerance Test

    a.   Purpose:  IV tolbutamide acutely stimu-
        lates insulin secretion.  The majority of
        pediatric patients with insulin secreting
        tumors have a much exaggerated response.

    b.   Method:  Administer tolbutamide 20 mg/kg
        (not to exceed 1 gm) intravenously over one
        minute.

    c.   Specimens:  Measure blood glucose and
        insulin at 0, 2, 5, 10, 20, 30, and 60
        minutes.

    d.   Interpretation:  Normal children exhibit
        a transient fall in blood glucose not ex-
        ceeding 50% of baseline.  Pediatric patients
        with insulinomas or other hyperinsulinemic
        states have prolonged, severe hypoglycemia
        in association with plasma insulin levels
        in excess of 100 microU/milliliter.  50%
        GLUCOSE SOLUTION SHOULD BE AT BEDSIDE.
        (Dose 1-2 ml/kg)

        Ref: J. Pediatric 82:558, 1973.
             Ann. Int. Med. 79:239, 1973.

8. Leucine Tolerance Test

    a.   Purpose:  To detect hypoglycemia secondary
        to leucine ingestion.

    b.   Method:  Leucine 150 mg/kg orally or 75 mg/
        kg IV is given over 2-5 minutes.

    c.   Specimens:  Measure plasma glucose and
        insulin at 0, 5, 15, 30, 45, 60 and 90
        minutes.

    d.   Interpretation:  Normal children have no
        change in blood glucose or insulin.  In
        the leucine sensitive patient, insulin
        rises acutely, followed by a decrease in
        blood sugar to 50% of baseline at 30 to
        45 minutes.  50% GLUCOSE SOLUTION SHOULD BE
        AT BEDSIDE. (Dose 1-2 ml/kg)

9. Tryptophan Load Test

    a.   Purpose:  To test tryptophan absorption
        and metabolism.  In Hartnup's disease and
        the blue diaper syndrome, tryptophan ab-
        sorption is blocked and indican (a metabo-
        lite of tryptophan produced by colonic
        bacteria) spills into the urine.  In
        pyridoxine deficiency and inherited
        abnormalities of the $B_6$ dependent enzyme,
        kynureninase, a tryptophan metabolite
        proximal to the metabolic block (xanthure-
        nic acid) spills into the urine.

b. Method:
   1) NPO for 12 hours.  Give L-tryptophan
      70 mg/kg/PO.
   2) To test for decreased kynureninase
      collect a 24 hour urine for xanthurenic
      acid.  Store urine in brown glass
      bottle at 4°C under 20 cc of toluene.
   3) To test for absorption abnormalities
      collect urine samples at 6, 12, and 24
      hours and test for indicanuria.
      Indicanuria:  Reagent: 2 gm FeCl3 in
      2 liter concentrated HCl.  Add 5 ml
      reagent to 4 ml of urine.  Mix then add
      2-3 ml chloroform.  Invert several times.
      A blue color in the chloroform indicates
      the presence of indican (indoxyl sulfate).

10. Phenylalanine Tolerance Test

   a. Purpose:  The detection of heterozygous
      carriers of the recessive gene for phenylketo-
      nuria.
   b. Method:  NPO for 12 hours.  Give 0.1 gm/kg
      of L-phenylalanine PO.
   c. Specimens:  Determine plasma phenylalanine
      concentration at 0, 1, 2 and 4 hours.
   d. Interpretation:  Heterozygote carriers in-
      crease to levels about twice those of normal
      controls at 1 and 2 hours.

      Ref:  Amer. J. Human Genet. 9:310, 1957.

B.  QUICK METHOD FOR PLASMA GLUCOSE

   Fill a heparinized microhematocrit tube with
   capillary blood and centrifuge it.  Using a micro-
   bulb, place 1 drop of the plasma on a Dextrostix.
   Allow to stand for 3 minutes.  Wash off with
   0.2 N (20%) sodium hydroxide and permit to dry.
   No change in color indicates less than 20 mg/100 ml;
   faint orange, 20 to 30 mg/100 ml; deep orange,
   greater than 40 mg/100 ml.  A standard curve can
   be prepared by using plasma of known glucose concentrations.  This value is an estimate and must
   be verified by a reliable laboratory method.

      Ref:  Pediat. Clin. N. Amer. 13:907, 1966.

C.  MISCELLANEOUS METABOLIC TESTS

   1.  The Ferric Chloride Reaction

      a. Principle:  Many compounds react with $Fe^{+++}$
         to form colored derivatives.  To interpret
         results remember the following:

     1) It is a relatively insensitive test
requiring relatively high concentrations of the reacting metabolite
(salicylate is an exception).

     2) Phosphate ions yield cloudy precipitates
which may mask positive result.

     3) Many compounds yield only a transient
color.

     4) Best done on <u>fresh</u> urine.

b. <u>Reagent</u>: The standard reagent is 10% FeCl₃.
Modified reagents used in specialized labs
are not considered here.

c. <u>Procedure</u>: Add 2 drops of reagent to 1 ml
of urine. Mix and observe color immediately and on standing.

d. <u>Interpretation</u>: (see chart next page)
<u>A negative result does not rule out disease.</u>

    <u>Ref</u>: Brit. Med. J. <u>2</u>:745, 1968
Selected Screening Tests for Genetic
Metabolic Disease; Thomas and Howell;
Yearbook Medical Publishers, 1973

2. <u>Semi-Quantitative Test for Calcium in Urine</u>

<u>Sulkowitch Test</u>
a. <u>Method</u>: To 5 ml of urine in a test tube
add 2 ml of Sulkowitch solution.
Compare resulting precipitate with the
opacity of a control (5 ml of test urine
and 2 ml of water). Note speed (3 to 30
seconds) of appearance and degree of den-
sity of solution. Results are recorded as
0, or 1-4+.

     Sulkowitch Solution
    Oxalic acid       2.5 gm
    Ammonium oxalate  2.5 gm
    Glacial acetic acid 5.0 ml
    Distilled water qs 150.0 ml

b. <u>Interpretation</u>: Zero test usually indicates
hypocalcemia (less than 7.5 mg%); 3-4+
test suggests hypercalcemia (more than 11
mg%). Certain factors other than disease
influence calcium concentration in the
urine, including specific gravity of the
urine, dietary calcium, and activity of
the patient. Test is of special value in
differentiating alkalotic from hypocalcemic
tetany, in diagnosing hypo- and hyperparathyroidism, and in managing vitamin D
dosage in refractory rickets and hypo-
parathyroidism.

INTERPRETATION OF FERRIC CHLORIDE REACTION

| Clinical Condition | Reacting Compound | Color Produced | |
|---|---|---|---|
| | | 10% FeCl3 | Phenistix |
| Normal | Phosphates | Brown to white precipitate which can obscure positive test. | |
| Phenylketonuria | Phenylpyruvic acid | Green, stable for few hours. | Grey-Green |
| Maple Syrup Urine Disease | Branch chain keto acids | Grey-green to green, stable. | |
| Histidinemia | Imidazole pyruvic acid | Dark green, stable indefinitely. | |
| Tyrosinemia | P-hydroxyphenyl pyruvic acid | Green, fades in seconds. | Green |
| Alkaptonuria | Homogentisic acid | Blue-green, fades in seconds. | |
| Oast house Disease | α-hydroxy butyric acid | Purple fading to red-brown | Green |
| Ketosis | Acetoacetic acid | Purple-red, fades in minutes. | |
| Direct Bilirubinemia | Bilirubin | Green, stable. | |

INTERPRETATION OF FERRIC CHLORIDE REACTION

| Clinical Condition | Reacting Compound | Color Produced | |
|---|---|---|---|
| | | 10% FeCl3 | Phenistix |
| Melanoma | Melanin | Gray precipitate-turning black. | |
| Carcinoid | 5-hydroxyindolacetic acid | Blue green | |
| Salicylate Ingestion | Salicylates | Purple, stable | Purple |
| PAS Ingestion | p-amino salicylic acid | Red-brown | Red-brown |
| Phenothiazine Ingestion | Phenothiazine derivatives | Blue-purple | Purple |
| Lysol Ingestion | Lysol | Green | |
| Antipyrine & Acetophenetidine Ingestion | Antipyrine & acetophenetidine derivatives | Cherry red | |
| L-Dopa Ingestion | L-Dopa metabolites | Green | |

Ref: <u>Parathyroid Glands and Metabolic
Bone Disease</u>; Albright, F. and
Reifenstein, E.C., Jr.; Baltimore:
Williams and Wilkins, 1948.

3. <u>Paper Spot Test for the Detection of Acid
Mucopolysaccharides in the Urine</u>

a. <u>Purpose</u>: Screening test for the mucopoly-
saccharidoses (e.g., Hunter, Hurler
Syndromes). A few false negatives and
false positives have been described.

b. <u>Method</u>: 5, 10, and 25 microliters of fresh
urine are placed as separate spots on a
piece of Whatman No. 1 filter paper.
(Note: Old urine, especially if infected,
will give false negatives.) A micropipette
should be used to add 5 microliters at a
time. Each application should be thoroughly
dry before the next is made. The paper
is then dipped in an aqueous solution
of 0.04% toluidine blue (buffered at pH
2.0 with Coleman's buffer tablets) for 1
minute using a petri dish, drained, and
rinsed in 95% ethyl alcohol.

c. <u>Interpretation</u>: A positive test is read
as a purple spot against a light blue
background. Normal urines will sometimes
give a faint rim of metachromatic material
around a blue spot.

4. <u>Porphyrinuria (Uroporphyrin and Coproporphyin)</u>

a. <u>Method</u>
   1) Acidify 5 ml of freshly voided urine
      with a few drops of glacial acetic
      acid to pH 4. Cap with thumb and shake
      vigorously to expel all $CO_2$.
   2) Add 15 ml of peroxide free ether
      (fresh anethesia ether is preferable),
      cap firmly with thumb and shake vigo-
      rously for 30 seconds. Pressure must
      be maintained with thumb until ether
      and urine layers separate.
   3) Transfer ether layer to a clean tube
      and add 5 ml of 1.5 N HCl. Then add
      0.25 ml of 0.1% iodine in 95% alcohol
      and shake vigorously for 30 seconds as
      in step 2.
   4) View original aqueous layer (Tube 1)
      and HCl layer (Tube 2) with a Wood's
      Lamp for the presence of fluorescence
      in a totally darkened room.

b. Interpretation
1) Uroporphyrins are ether-insoluble, and cause fluorescence in aqueous fraction of tube 1. They are never present in normal urine. Marked uroporphyrinuria occurs almost exclusively in congenital acute and chronic forms of porphyria where coproporphyrins are usually increased also. If tests for porphobilinogen is also positive, the condition is probably acute hepatic porphyria.
2) Coproporphyrins cause fluorescence in the HCl layer of tube 2.

Traces of coproporphyrins are present in normal urine, usually in amounts too small to give a strongly positive reaction. Coproporphyrinuria without uroporphyrinuria occurs in conditions associated with:
a) Increased hematopoietic activity; sickle cell and other hemolytic anemias, pernicious anemia after treatment, hemorrhage, etc.
b) Hepatic insufficiency: infectious hepatitis, atresia or obstruction of biliary system, cirrhosis, etc.
c) Toxic interference with hemoglobin synthesis (lead, arsenic, mercury intoxication, etc.)
d) Miscellaneous: poliomyelitis (particularly bulbar), rheumatic fever, acute and severe febrile illnesses, methemoglobinemia, carbon monoxide poisoning, and idiopathic coproporphyrinuria.

A strongly positive test in HCl is usually indicative of acute lead poisoning, although it may also be seen in hepatitis. A weakly positive test is seen in mild or resolving lead poisoning and in the other conditions mentioned above.

When available, determination of free erythrocyte protoporphyrin levels on capillary blood is the recommended method for screening for lead poisoning.

Ref: Ped. 52:303, 1973

| ARBITRARY SCALE OF FLUORESCENCE INTENSITY OF COPROPORPHYRIN SOLUTIONS | | |
|---|---|---|
| Arbitrary Scale | Color | Approximate Quantitative Equivalent of Coproporphyrin |
| 0 | Blue-violet | <0.1 micrograms/ml of urine |
| + | Faint blue-orange | <0.1 micrograms/ml of urine |
| ++ | Blue-orange | <0.2 micrograms/ml of urine |
| +++ | Orange-red | <0.5 micrograms/ml of urine |
| ++++ | Deep orange-red | >0.5 micrograms/ml of urine |

5. <u>Porphobilinogen (Watson and Schwartz)</u>

   a. <u>Purpose:</u>  Found in exacerbation of acute intermittent hepatic porphyria.
   b. <u>Reagents:</u>
      1) Ehrlich's aldehyde reagent.
      2) Sodium acetate, saturated solution:
             100 gm Na acetate
             100 ml H2O
      3) Chloroform.
   c. <u>Method:</u>
      1) 5 ml of freshly voided urine is added to 5 ml of Ehrlich's adehyde reagent and shaken for 30 seconds.
      2) Saturated aqueous sodium acetate is added to bring to pH of 4-5.  If the solution is red at this point then porphobilinogen, urobilinogen or certain indole compounds are present.
      3) If any red pigment is present then extraction with 10 ml of chloroform to remove urobilinogen is performed repeatedly until no more red pigment is extracted by the chloroform.
      4) If any red pigment remains in the aqueous phase it is extracted with 5 ml of n-butanol.  After extraction with the n-butanol, any red pigment remaining in the aqueous phase is porphobilinogen.

6. <u>Alternate Test for Urine Porphobilinogin (Hoesch test)</u>

   a. <u>Reagents:</u>  Modified Ehrlich's reagent 20 grams p-dimethylamino benzaldehyde diluted to 1000 ml with 6 N HCl.  This is not the Ehrlich's aldehyde used for Watson-Schwartz.

b.  Method:
    1.  Add 2 drops of fresh urine to 3 ml of
        modified Ehrlich's reagent.
c.  Results:  Instantaneous cherry red color
    indicates significant urinary porphobilinogen.
    Urobilinogen does not give false positive
    results.  Sensitivity of the Hoesch test
    is equal to the Watson Schwartz.

    Ref:  Clin. Chem. 20: 1438, 1974

## T E S T S   O F   U P P E R

## G A S T R O I N T E S T I N A L   F U N C T I O N

1. <u>Augmented Histamine Test</u>

    A. <u>Purpose</u>: To aid in the diagnosis of certain
       hyper or hypoacidity states (<u>e.g.</u> Zollinger-
       Ellison Syndrome) by measuring the gastric
       secretion of HCl in a basal state and fol-
       lowing stimulation by histamine. The
       variability of the results in children makes
       it unreliable in diagnosis of peptic ulcer
       disease.

    B  Method:
       1) Patients fast beginning at midnight be-
          fore the test. Infants younger than one
          year need fast for only 4-6 hours.
       2) A radio-opaque tube is passed into the
          stomach and the position of the tube is
          adjusted under fluoroscopy so that the
          tip is in the pylorus.
       3) The patient lies on his right side or
          supine or sits for the remainder of the
          test.
       4) Fasting gastric secretion is aspirated
          and discarded.
       5) Gastric secretions are then collected by
          manual suction every 15 minutes for one
          hour and saved in an iced container.
          This represents basal secretion.
       6) Betazol (Histalog, Lilly), 1.0 mg/kg, is
          injected sub-Q. Minor side reactions may
          be prevented by prior administration of
          diphenhydramine.
       7) Four 15 minute samples of gastric secretion
          are again collected and saved in an iced
          container. This represents post stimulation
          gastric secretion.
       8) Each 15 minute sample is measured for pH,
          volume, and titratable acidity.

    C. <u>Normal Values</u>:
       Gastroenterology <u>52</u>:1101, 1967.
       Am. J. Dig. Dis. <u>14</u>:404, 1969.

2. <u>Semi-Quantitative Analysis of Duodenal Secretions
   for Activity of Pancreatic Trypsin</u>

    A. <u>Duodenal Intubation</u>: Chilled duodenal secre-
       tions are collected in the following manner:

1) Pass a Levin or similar tube into the
   stomach.  If a weighted tube is used, the
   weight should have the same diameter as the
   tube.  In larger children a Miller-Abbott
   tube may be used.  If possible a double
   lumen tube should be used to avoid contamination with gastric contents.
2) Position patient on right side and place
   tube on gravity drainage.
3) At intervals of 1/2 to 1 hour check the
   drainage for color and pH, advancing tube
   until fluid is bile stained or alkaline.

B. <u>Examination of Duodenal Fluid</u>:  Make serial
   dilutions of the duodenal fluid.

| Tube | Duodenal Fluid | 5% NaHCO$_3$ | Final Dilution |
|---|---|---|---|
| 1 | .5 ml | 5.75 ml | 1:12-1/2 |
| 2 | 2 ml from tube 1 | 2 ml | 1:25 |
| 3 | 2 ml from tube 2 | 2 ml | 1:50 |
| 4 | 2 ml from tube 3 | 2 ml | 1:100 |
| 5 | 2 ml from tube 4 | 2 ml | 1:200 |
| 6 | 2 ml from tube 5 | 2 ml | 1:400 |
| 7 | 2 ml from tube 6 | 2 ml | 1:800 |
| 8 | 2 ml from tube 7 | 2 ml | 1:1600 |
| 9 | 2 ml from tube 8 | 2 ml | 1:3200 |
| 10 | none | 2 ml | control |

Discard 2 ml from tube 9.  To each tube add
2 ml of 7-1/2% gelatin.  Place tubes in incu-
bator at 37°C for 1 hour, then refrigerate
until tube 10 (control) is solid (overnight
advised).

Tryptic activity indicated by liquefaction of
gelatin persisting after refrigeration.

C. <u>Interpretation</u>:  Normal activity indicated by
   liquefaction through dilution 1:400 (tubes
   1-6 or greater).  Borderline activity indicated
   by liquefaction in tubes 1-5 only (marasmus,
   etc.).  Pancreatic deficiency <u>is</u> suggested by
   liquefaction in tubes 1-3 only (cystic fibrosis,
   obstruction of pancreatic duct, etc.).

<u>NOTE</u>:  If duodenal juice is contaminated with
gastric secretions the test is invalid.

3. <u>Mono and Disaccharide Absorption Tests</u>

   A. <u>Purpose</u>: To diagnose malabsorption of a specific carbohydrate by measuring the change in blood glucose following an oral dose of the carbohydrate in question.

   B. <u>Method</u>:
      1) The patient fasts 4-6 hours prior to test.
      2) The test carbohydrate (lactose, sucrose, maltose, glucose, galactose) is given orally or by gastric tube in a dose of 2.0 gm/kg as a 10% solution (maximum dose of 100 gms.). For maltose the dose is 1.0 gm/kg.
      3) Serum glucose is measured prior to the carbohydrate dose and at 15, 30, 60, and 90 minutes following the dose.
      4) The number and character of the stools, the stool pH, and the results of a Clini-test determination for reducing substances should be noted on all stools passed during the test and for 8 hours after the test is completed.

   C. <u>Interpretation</u>:
      1) A rise in the blood glucose level of 25 mg/100 ml over the fasting level within the test period is considered normal. An increase of 20 to 25 mg/100 ml is questionable. Increases of less than 20 mg/100 ml are abnormal and suggest mal-absorption of the test carbohydrate.
      2) Malabsorption is also suggested if during the test or subsequent 8 hour period one notes:
         1. The onset of diarrhea
         2. Stool pH of 6.0 or less
         3. Greater than 0.25% reducing substances (Clinitest) in the stool. <u>Note</u>: Sucrose is not a reducing substance.
         4. Crampy abdominal pain or abdominal distention.

4. <u>D-Xylose Test</u>

   A. <u>Purpose</u>: To evaluate the integrity of the duodenojejunal intestinal mucosa by measuring the absorption of an oral dose of D-xylose. Either the elevation in serum concentration or the % urinary excretion of xylose may be used to quantitate D-xylose absorption. Absorption is independent of bile salts, pancreatic exo-crine secretions, and intestinal mucosal

disaccharidases. The test is unreliable in
patients with edema, renal disease, delayed
gastric emptying and severe diarrhea.

B. Method:
  1) Preparation - Older children fast for 8
    hours prior to the test; younger infants
    need fast for only 4-6 hours.
  2) Test Dose - D-xylose in a dose of 0.5
    gm/kg (with a maximum of 5 grams) in a 5%
    water solution is given orally or via a
    gastric tube. Placement in the duodenum
    minimizes error caused by delayed gastric
    emptying.
  3) Measurement of Urinary Excretion -
    Patient voids and all urine for 5 hours is
    collected. Adequate urine flow is insured
    by supplementary oral or IV fluid. The
    quantity of xylose is determined colori-
    metrically.

    Normal Values: 5 hour urinary excretion
    of 25% or greater of the administered dose
    is normal for children over 6 months.
    Values between 15 and 25% are questionable.
    Urinary excretion of less than 15% is ab-
    normal. In infants less than 6 months
    values below 10% are considered abnormal.

  4) Measurement of Serum Concentration -
    Serum samples for determination of xylose
    concentration are obtained in fasting state
    and at 30, 60, 90, and 120 minutes following
    the xylose dose.

    Normal Values: A normal response is asso-
    ciated with a serum level exceeding 20 mg/
    100 ml in any of the post absorptive
    specimens.

    Ref: New Eng. J. Med. 268: 1441, 1963.
         Pediat. 48:59, 1971.
         JAMA 186:517, 1963.

5. Quantitative Fecal Fat

A. Purpose: Quantitative Determination of
fecal fat excretion to aid in diagnosis or
management of the fat malabsorption syndromes.

B. Method:
  1) The patient is given a diet with a rela-
    tively constant percentage of fat for 3 days
    prior to the collection period. Note:
    Regular ward diets containing approximately
    35% of calories as fat are adequate.

2) A charcoal marker (3 tablets for children under 6 years and 6 tablets for children over 6 years of age) is given at the beginning of the collection period and again 72 hours later.

3) All stools passed from the appearance of the 1st marker until the appearance of the 2nd marker should be saved in a pre-weighed can and refrigerated. Note: In patients with diarrhea the use of markers is unnecessary. A simple 72 hour time collection is adequate.

4) Total fecal fatty acid content is determined.

C. Interpretation  Normal fecal fat excretion on a diet composed of approximately 35% fat is less than 5 gm/24 hours. Severe anorexia with decreased caloric intake will result in falsely low values so that the percentage fecal excretion of fat will be a more accurate index of fat malabsorption.

Ref: Ped. 46:690, 1970.

6. Bromsulphalein Test

This test should be performed fasting or after a carbohydrate meal since fat in the serum interferes with the estimation of the color. The test is invalid in the presence of marked jaundice.

A. Procedure:
1) Draw control sample.
2) Inject 5 mg/kg of body weight over a 5 minute period. (Caution: BSP in subcutaneous tissue is very irritating.)
3) Draw 45 minute sample from vein other than that used in #2.
4) Serious anaphylactoid reactions have been reported (although rare). A careful allergic history should be obtained.

B. Normal: First 2 weeks = 25% retention. Then 5% retention or less.

CARDIOLOGY

A. CARDIAC CYCLE
(see illustration on next page)

B. ELECTROCARDIOGRAPHY

1. <u>Terminology</u> (see illustration on next page)

The <u>P wave</u> is the result of atrial depolarization. The <u>QRS complex</u> is the result of
ventricular depolarization. Within this
complex the <u>Q wave</u> is the initial negative wave,
the <u>R wave</u> the first positive wave, and the
<u>S wave</u> a negative wave following the R wave.
When there is only a negative component to the
QRS complex, it is called a <u>QS wave</u>. <u>R' and
S' waves</u> refer to a second positive and negative
wave following R and S waves, respectively, in
the same QRS complex. <u>ST segment</u> refers to
that segment between the end of the QRS complex
and the beginning of the T wave. The <u>T wave</u> is
due to ventricular repolarization, which creates
a constant wave following the QRS complex,
usually of lower amplitude and longer duration.
The <u>U wave</u> is a small wave occasionally seen
following the T wave. U waves may be noted in
electrocardiograms of normal adolescents or in
individuals having hypokalemia. The <u>PR interval</u>
is measured from the beginning of the P wave
to the beginning of the QRS complex. The <u>QT
interval</u> is measured from the beginning of the
QRS complex to the end of the T wave.

2. <u>Placement and Meaning of Leads</u>

a. <u>Bipolar Leads:</u>
Lead   I: Right Arm - Left Arm
Lead  II: Right Arm - Left Leg
Lead III: Left Arm - Left leg

b. <u>Unipolar Leads:</u>
aVR: Right Arm
aVL: Left Arm
aVF: Left Foot

c. <u>Precordial Leads:</u>
V1  : 4th RICS at RSB
V2  : 4th LICS at LSB
V3  : Halfway between V2 + V4
V4  : 5th LICS at MCL
V5  : 5th LICS at AAL
V6  : 5th LICS at MAL
V3R : V3 on right chest
V7  : Posterior axillary line.
(use if no Q wave found in V6)

62

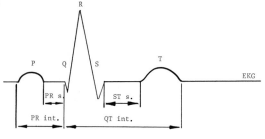

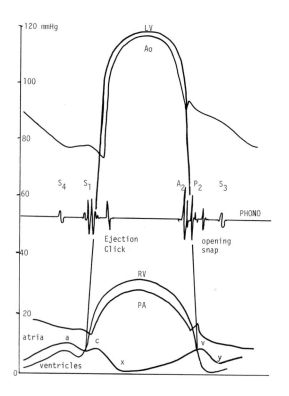

3. Rate

Rate may be obtained by multiplying by 20 the
number of complexes between two vertical lines
(3 seconds) at the top of the strip. If rate
is slow or irregular, a more accurate reflection
of rate is obtained by multiplying by 10 the
number of complexes between three vertical lines
(6 seconds). Record atrial and ventricular
rates when AV block is present.

### Heart Rate at Various Ages

| Age | Heart Rate Mean | Range |
|---|---|---|
| 0-24 hours | 145 | 80-200 |
| 1- 7 days | 138 | 100-188 |
| 8-30 days | 162 | 125-188 |
| 1- 3 months | 161 | 115-215 |
| 3- 6 months | 149 | 100-215 |
| 6-12 months | 147 | 100-188 |
| 1- 3 years | 130 | 80-188 |
| 3- 5 years | 105 | 68-150 |
| 5- 8 years | 105 | 68-150 |
| 8-12 years | 88 | 51-125 |
| 12-16 years | 83 | 38-125 |

Modified from Ziegler, R.F.:
Electrocardiographic Studies in Normal
Infants and Children, Springfield, Ill:
Charles C. Thomas, 1951.

4. Rhythm

The entire strip should be examined to ex-
clude abnormalities of rhythm.

5. P Waves

a. Atrial Enlargement
   1) RAE suggested by spiked "P Pulmonale"
      type P waves higher than 2.5 mm and
      best seen in L-2 and aVR (ꓥ).
   2) LAE suggested by plateau or notched
      "P Mitrale" type P waves longer than
      0.08 seconds (ꟽ).
   3) McCruz Index - P/PR segment ratio has
      been used to indicate atrial enlarge-
      ment in the absence of A-V block. A
      ratio less than 1 suggest RAE and
      greater than 1.6 suggests LAE.
   4) Terminal and deep inversion of the P
      wave in V1-2 suggests LAE especially
      when the P wave is prolonged (ꟽ).

# EINTHOVEN TRIANGLE

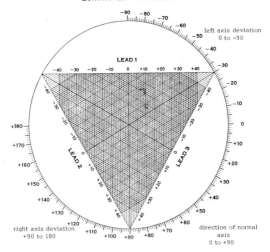

# FRONTAL AXIS

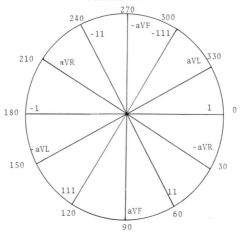

b. Atrial Inversion
   1) True Dextrocardia: characterized by
      a P vector oriented to the right,
      inferior and anterior.  The P wave is
      inverted in L-I and upright in aVR.  The
      left precordial leads have a diminished
      V6 type progression.
   2) Technical Dextrocardia: same as true
      dextrocardia except precordial leads
      are normal.

c. Abnormal Rhythm
   1) Coronary sinus rhythm: shortened to
      normal PR interval with negative P in
      L-2, L-3, aVF and upright in V6.
   2) Left atrial rhythm: varying P config-
      urations in limb leads depending on
      site of origin (high, low or mid);
      however, frequently negative in L-2,
      L-3, aVF and always negative in V6.
      Dome and Dart configuration diagnostic
      of left atrial rhythm with the dome
      representing left atrium and dart the
      right atrium.  Best seen in L-2 and
      V1.

6. PR Interval

Maximal PR Interval (Longest PR in Any Limb Lead)

| Age | \multicolumn{6}{c}{Rate} | | | | | |
|---|---|---|---|---|---|---|
| | -70 | 71-90 | 91-110 | 111-130 | 131-150 | 151- |
| Under 1 month | | | .11 | .11 | .11 | .11 |
| 1-9 months | | | .14 | .13 | .12 | .11 |
| 10-24 months | | | .15 | .14 | .14 | .10 |
| 3-5 years | | .16 | .16 | .16 | | |
| 6-13 years | .18 | .18 | .16 | .16 | | |

7. QRS Complex

   a. QRS Complex: Measure longest complex in any
      lead.  Relatively independent of age and
      rate.
   b. Q Wave: qR in V3R or V1, never normal after
      24 hours of age.  If of sufficient depth
      and width, may be significant in any lead
      even in the pediatric age group for ischemia
      and/or hypertrophy.

8. QRS Axis

   See preceding page for calculation of mean
   electrical axis.

### QRS Axis At Various Ages

| Age | QRS Axis Mean | Range |
|---|---|---|
| 0-24 hours | 137° | 70-205° |
| 1- 7 days | 125° | 75-185° |
| 8-30 days | 108° | 30-190° |
| 1- 3 months | 75° | 25-125° |
| 3- 6 months | 65° | 30- 96° |
| 6-12 months | 65° | 10-115° |
| 1- 3 years | 55° | 6-108° |
| 3- 5 years | 62° | 20-105° |
| 5- 8 years | 65° | 16-112° |
| 8-12 years | 62° | 15-112° |
| 12-16 years | 65° | 20-116° |

Modified from Ziegler, R.F.: Electrocardio-graphic Studies in Normal Infants and Children, Springfield, Ill.: Charles C. Thomas, 1951.

9. QT Interval

### Normal QT Interval

| Rate | Mean | +2 S.D. |
|---|---|---|
| 55 | .42 | .36-.48 |
| 65 | .39 | .34-.44 |
| 75 | .36 | .31-.41 |
| 85 | .34 | .29-.38 |
| 95 | .32 | .27-.36 |
| 110 | .30 | .25-.34 |
| 130 | .27 | .23-.31 |
| 160 | .25 | .21-.28 |
| 200 | .22 | .18-.25 |

10. QTc (Corrected QT Interval)

$$QTc = \sqrt{\frac{QT\ measured}{cycle\ length}} = \text{not greater than } 0.425$$

See next page for Nomogram.

11. T Wave

Inversion in I: Normal for first 24 hours only. Dextrocardia or myo-cardial disturbance.
II. Myocardial or pericardial disturbance.
III. Normal.

# RATE CORRECTION OF Q-T INTERVAL

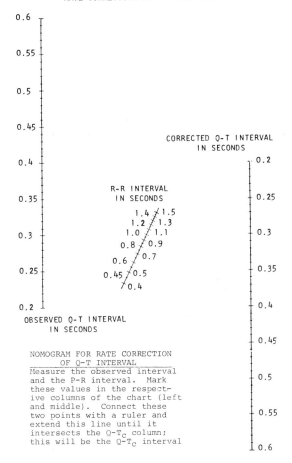

CORRECTED Q-T INTERVAL
IN SECONDS

R-R INTERVAL
IN SECONDS

OBSERVED Q-T INTERVAL
IN SECONDS

NOMOGRAM FOR RATE CORRECTION
OF Q-T INTERVAL
Measure the observed interval
and the P-R interval. Mark
these values in the respect-
ive columns of the chart (left
and middle). Connect these
two points with a ruler and
extend this line until it
intersects the Q-T$_C$ column;
this will be the Q-T$_C$ interval

| | T Wave inverted or bi-phasic in over 50% of individuals until age: | May be normal until age: |
|---|---|---|
| V1 | 12 years | 17 years |
| V2 | 8 years | 13 years |
| V3 | 3 years | 10 years |
| V4 | 24 hours | 5 years |
| V5 | - | 24 hours |
| V6 | - | 24 hours |

12: Ventricular Hypertrophy

    a. Right Ventricular Hypertrophy (any of below, singly or in combination):
1) RV1 >20 mm (>29 under 1 month)
2) SV6 >7 mm (>14 under 1 month)
3) R/S V1 >2 after 6 months
4) Upright TV1 after 4 days
5) qR in V1 or V3R.

    b. Left Ventricular Hypertrophy (any of below, singly or in combination):
1) RV6 >25 mm (>20 mm in 1st year)
2) SV1 >20 mm
3) R/S in V1 <0.8 under 1 year
        <0.2 1-5 years
        <0.1 6-13 years
4) 2° T wave inversion in V5 or V6
5) Q>3 mm in V5 or V6.

    c. Combined Ventricular Hypertrophy:
1) Direct signs of right + left
2) RVH and
   a) q 2 mm or more in V6
   b) sizable RV 6
   c) T inversion in V6
3) LVH and
   a) sizable RV1
   b) RAD
4) "Normal" EKG with cardiomegaly

## 13.  Overload Patterns

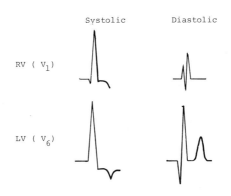

|  | Systolic | Diastolic |
|---|---|---|
| RV ( $V_1$ ) | | |
| LV ( $V_6$ ) | | |

## 14.  Useful Normal R + S Wave Values

| | AGE | R (mm) | S (mm) | R (% R+S) | R/S RATIO | V.A.T. (sec.) |
|---|---|---|---|---|---|---|
| **V-1** | ‹ I MONTH | 4 - 28 (13) | 0 - 15 (6) | 40 - 90 (60) | .66 - 9.0 (1.2) | .005 - .030 (.02) |
| | ‹ I YEAR | 1 - 19 (10) | 0 - 18 (6) | 40 - 80 (50) | .66 - 4.0 (1.0) | .010 - .030 (.02) |
| | 1 - 8 YRS. | 1 - 19 (7) | 0 - 25 (12) | 10 - 60 (35) | .11 - 1.2 (.54) | .000 - .025 (.015) |
| | 8 - 16 YRS. | 1 - 16 (4) | 3 - 24 (15) | 10 - 50 (30) | .11 - 1.0 (.43) | .000 - .030 (.020) |
| **V-2** | ‹ I MONTH | 7 - 31 (19) | 3 - 35 (19) | | | |
| | ‹ I YEAR | 7 - 28 (17) | 3 - 35 (19) | | | |
| | 1 - 8 YRS. | 1 - 31 (14) | 7 - 39 (21) | | | |
| | 8 - 16 YRS. | 1 - 19 (10) | 7 - 39 (19) | | | |
| **V-5** | ‹ I MONTH | 2 - 34 (14) | 0 - 18 (6) | | | .005 - .025 (.02) |
| | ‹ I YEAR | 6 - 26 (18) | 0 - 15 (2) | | | .015 - .040 (.025) |
| | 1 - 8 YRS. | 10 - 38 (20) | 0 - 9 (1) | | | .020 - .040 (.030) |
| | 8 - 16 YRS. | 6 - 34 (16) | 0 - 9 (1) | | | .020 - .040 (.035) |

★

|  | R/S V5 R/S VI |
|---|---|
| 1 - 6 MONTHS | .2 - 6 |
| 1/2 - 2 YEARS | .4 - 8 |
| 2 - 6 YEARS | .5 - 10 |
| 6 - 10 YEARS | 1.0 - 20 |
| 10 - 16 YEARS | 1.5 - 45 |

RVH = BELOW MINIMUM
LVH = ABOVE MAXIMUM

15. <u>Bundle Branch Block</u>

    a. <u>Incomplete</u>:
       1) Longest QRS <0.10 when associated
          with slurred QRS or RSR prime.
    b. <u>Complete</u>: Longest QRS >0.10
       1) LBBB:
          a) LAD
          b) R in I tall + late. T in I
             sharply inverted.
          c) S in V1 and V2 wide.
       2) RBBB:
          a) RAD
          b) S in I wide and deep. T in I
             upright.
          c) S in V5 and V6 wide.

16. <u>Digitalis</u>

    a. <u>Effect</u>:
       1) QTc interval shortened.
       2) T waves depressed, then inverted.
       3) ST segment depressed.
       4) PR interval prolonged.
       5) Sinus arrhythmia.
    b. <u>Toxicity</u>:
       1) Various degrees of AV block.
       2) Bradycardia.
       3) Arrhythmias of any type, commonly
          atrial in children, ventricular in
          adults.

17. <u>Electrolyte Disturbances</u>

    a. <u>Hyperkalemia</u>: Serial EKG's in an individual
       can be correlated with serum K+.
       1) T wave: tall, tented, narrow.
       2) PR, QRS, and QT lengthened. QRS may
          prolong so it blends with T to
          produce diphasic curve.
       3) P wave widened and flattened,
          finally disappearing.
       4) R wave widened and flattened.
       5) S wave deepened.
       6) Ectopic rhythms and intraventricular
          block.

<u>NOTE</u> These effects are enhanced by Na+ or
Ca++ depletion.

    b. <u>Intracellular Potassium Depletion</u> (with
       intracellular Na+ excess): Fair cor-
       relation with serum K+.
       1) QT lengthened (due to broad, flat T
          wave).

    2) T wave flattened or inverted.
    3) ST segment depressed.
    4) U wave prominent.

    NOTE: These effects are enhanced by digitalis intoxication. It is probably the ratio of extracellular K/intracellular K that determines EKG changes. Concurrent calcium and sodium changes also play a role.

  c. Hypocalcemia: QT interval lengthened (due to long ST segment).
  d. Hypercalcemia:
    1) QT interval sometimes shortened (due to shortened ST segment).
    2) Myocardial irritability increased: PVCs, ventricular tachycardia.

C. ECHOCARDIOGRAPHY

  1. Scan Technique (See diagram page 74)

    An ultrasonic probe (3-5 MHz) is placed over the fourth LICS and directed posteriorly. The unique M-configuration of the anterior mitral leaflet, the essential landmark of standardization, is located in this position. A cardiac scan from the apex to the base of the heart can be performed by angling the transducer inferolaterally towards the apex. (Position 1) Echoes return from the left ventricular side of the interventricular septum (IVS) and the posterior left ventricular wall (LVW). The IVS and posterior LVW approach one another during systole and recede during diastole. Measurement of these phasic dimensions are used to calculate an ejection fraction. Standardization of this area is assured by inclusion of a small portion of the mitral apparatus. It may not be possible to record the right ventricle (RV) because of its flattened shape and trabeculated anatomy.

    When the transducer is slowly angled cranially, the prominent M-shaped anterior mitral leaflet (AML) motion will come into view. Careful manipulation of the probe will reveal the posterior mitral leaflet (PML) moving in the opposite direction during diastole and merging with the anterior leaflet during systole (Position 2).

The maximum excursion of the mitral valve
and its closing velocity are recorded when
the transducer is further rotated cranio-
medially into Position 3.  In this area
the transducer beam transects an atrioven-
tricular area.  The motion of this area is
characterized by low amplitude excursions
in contrast to the high amplitude rhythmic
motion of the posterior LVW seen in positions 1 and 2.  When the transducer is
again rotated cranially and slightly
medially, the anterior and posterior parallel moving walls of the aorta (Ao) are
visualized (Position 4).  The anterior
aortic echo is at the same depth as the IVS
while the posterior aortic reflection is
in continuity with the anterior mitral
leaflet.  The aortic valve (AV) leaflet
will be noted to separate during systole
and merge during diastole, forming a box
pattern during systole within the parallel walls of the aorta.  The left atrium
(LA) visualizes just posterior to the
aorta.

2.  Indications for Echocardiography:

a.  Diagnostic for the following defects:
    1)  Prolapsed mitral leaflet
    2)  Mitral stenosis
    3)  Idiopathic hypertrophic
        subaortic stenosis
    4)  Tetralogy of Fallot
    5)  Atrioventricular canal
    6)  Ostium primum defect
    7)  Hypoplastic left heart syndrome
    8)  Pericardial or pleural effusion
    9)  Atrial tumors

b.  Very helpful for:
    1)  Aortic insufficiency
    2)  Transposition of the great vessels
    3)  Truncus ateriosus
    4)  Diastolic overload of the right ventricle
    5)  Hypoplastic right heart syndrome
    6)  Single ventricle
    7)  Ebstein's anomaly
    8)  Subvalvular aortic stenosis
    9)  Double outlet right ventricle
    10) Prosthetic valves

    c. For serial evaluations of:
       1) Dilatation
       2) Hypertrophy
       3) LV function
       4) Dyskinetic areas

3. Normal Values

   Reference:

   Echocardiography; Feigenbaum; Lea and Febiger,
   Philadelphia; 1972

   Circulation 47: 108, 1973

   Circulation 48: 1221, 1973

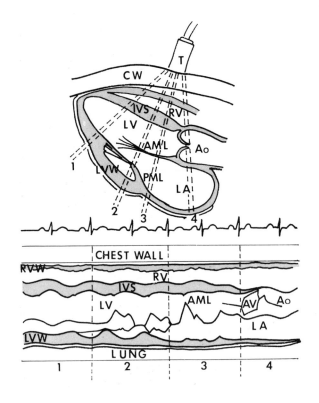

X-RAY CONTOUR OF HEART

Right Anterior Oblique     Left Anterior Oblique     Antero-Posterior

NORMAL INTRACARDIAC PRESSURES

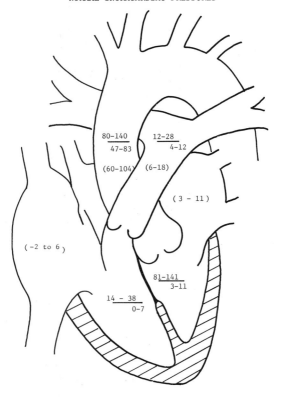

$$\frac{80-140}{47-83}$$

(60-104)

$$\frac{12-28}{4-12}$$

(6-18)

( 3 - 11 )

( -2 to 6 )

$$\frac{81-141}{3-11}$$

$$\frac{14 - 38}{0-7}$$

Normal pressures based on normal patients 2 months to 20 years of age.

Systolic/Diastolic with ± 2 S.D. range
(Mean Pressure)

ENDOCRINOLOGY

1. Thyroid Tests*

   Normal values must be obtained from the individual
   laboratories since methods and data presentation
   may vary.

   Ref: J. Pediat. 82: 1, 1973
        J. Clin. Endocrinol. Metab. 34: 884, 1972

   a. *Thyroxine by Column ($T_4(C)$)

      Normal values 2.9-6.4 micrograms/100 ml
      (as iodine, $T_4$ is 63.5 per cent iodine by weight)

   b. *Thyroxine by Displacement ($T_4(D)$)

      These results are not influenced by inorganic
      iodine or by organic non-thyroxine iodine
      contamination.

      Normal values      5.1-11.5 micrograms/100 ml
         Cord            7.3-17.7 micrograms/100 ml
         24 hrs.         16.4-27.7 micrograms/100 ml
         48 hrs.         19.8-24.0 micrograms/100 ml

      Ref: J. Clin. Invest. 52: 1195, 1973

   c. *Free Thyroxine ($FT_4$)

      Measures the non-protein-bound (dialyzable,
      "metabolically active" $T_4$) in contrast to
      $T_4(C)$ and $T_4(D)$ which measure all available $T_4$.

      Normal Values 1.0-2.1 nanograms/100 ml.

   d. *Triiodothyronine by Radioimmunoassay ($T_3(RIA)$)

         Normal values:

         Newborn  30-100 nanograms/100 ml.
         More than one week 50-220 nanograms/100 ml.

   e. *Thyroid Stimulating Hormone (TSH) by
      Radioimmunoassay

      This test is very dependent on the method used.
      Often one cannot differentiate abnormally low
      values from normal, since up to 40% of normals
      may have values below the lower limit of
      detectability of the assay.

      Normal values <2-10 microunits/ml

*Routinely available from Bioscience Laboratories,
Van Nuys, California.

f. *Thyroxine Binding Globulin (TBG)

Measures the binding capacity for $T_4$. Increases with estrogens and decreases with androgens, nephrotic syndrome, protein losing enteropathy. Occasionally, congenital deficiency occurs.

Normal values: 10-26 micrograms $T_4$ bound/100 ml

g. *Thyroid Antibodies

Normal values:
        Anti-thyroglobulin  <1:16
        Anti-microsomal     <1:4

May be variably elevated in thyrotoxicosis, and subacute and chronic thyroiditis.

h. Protein Bound Iodine (PBI)

Bioscience Laboratories no longer routinely performs this test which measures all iodinated proteins in serum.

Normal values: 4-8 micrograms/100 ml.

i. Radioactive Iodine Uptake (RAIU)

Measures uptake of $^{131}I$ by the thyroid gland - microcuries of $^{131}I$ are given by mouth and uptake is measured at 4 and 24 hours. The activity in the thyroid is expressed as a percentage of the total dose of radioactivity administered. The values for this test vary greatly with the dietary iodine content and recent normal values are lower than previous values.

Normal values:
        4 hours up to 12 per cent
        24 hours    ∿6-33 per cent

j. Perchlorate discharge test

Administer 10 mg/kg oral potassium perchlorate 60 to 120 minutes after tracer dose of $^{131}I$. Test is positive (organification "block") if more than 10% of the accumulated iodine is released.

*Routinely available from Bioscience Laboratories, Van Nuys, California.

k.  Thyroid scan

Most useful isotope is $^{99m}Tc$ - pertechnetate because it is short lived and reduces the radiation dose to the patient (compared to $^{131}I$.) It is especially helpful in localizing ectopic thyroid tissue.

l.  Thyrotropin-Releasing Hormone Test (TRH)

Measures pituitary TSH reserve. A negative test is confirmatory for hyperthyroidism. TRH (synthetic) is injected intravenously (3-6 micrograms/kg) and serum collected for 1.5 to 2 hours (peak usually 10 to 20 minutes after injection).

Normal values:  at least doubling of baseline values

m.  Tri-iodothyronine ($T_3$) Suppression

When $T_3$ is given, TSH secretion is suppressed unless thyroid gland is functioning autonomously, e.g., thyrotoxicosis, hyperfunctioning nodule.

Method:  After baseline RAIU, administer $T_3$, 125 micrograms/day, for 7 days and repeat RAIU on days 6 and 7. Normally the RAIU falls to 40% of the control.

2.  Toluidine Blue Stain for Chromatin Pattern of Buccal Smear

a.  Preparation of Smear from Buccal Mucous Membrane:  The mucous membrane is wiped with saline soaked gauze to remove bacteria and debris which might interfere with the interpretation of the smear. A metal spatula with a rounded end but a sharp angled scraping edge is used to scrape the buccal mucous membrane with mild to moderate pressure such that a small but visible amount of whitish material is seen at the end of the spatula base. The scraping is "dabbed" onto the center of a slide (not albuminized), spread thinly and evenly, and immediately inserted into the fixative.

b.  Fixative:  95% ethyl alcohol. The slides may remain in the fixative for 1 to 2 hours.

c. Staining

Toluidine blue    - 4 minutes

Distilled H$_2$0    - 2 dips

95% Ethanol    - 12 dips

100% Ethanol    - 12 dips

Xylene + mount

d. Reading of the Smear: Count 100 good quality cells under oil immersion. In the female, more than 20% of cells show a darkly stained chromatin mass adjacent to the nuclear membrane. Often a chromatin mass is seen within the nucleus which is not at the periphery. A cell is considered positive, however, only when a mass is noted against the nuclear membrane. In the male most cells show no mass at the nuclear membrane. Occasionally an ill-defined mass is seen but the percentage should not exceed 2%.

In females with the trisomy XXX syndrome and in males with trisomy XXXY "double" chromatin masses are seen and one patient has been described with four separate peripheral nuclear chromatin bodies.

e. Control: In order to be sure that the stain is proper, a female control buccal smear is run through with each group of unknowns. The easy visualization of the chromatin mass in the female control smear is a test of the adequacy of the staining technique.

3. Tests for Estrogen and Gonadotropins (LH + FSH)

a. Vaginal Smears

As children often have very little secretion, it is sometimes necessary to have a drop of salt solution in a pipette before attempting to aspirate the vagina. The aspirated secretion is immediately spread thinly upon a slide and immediately fixed for 1 minute in a mixture of ether and 95% alcohol in equal parts, allowing no drying lest distortion of the cells and their staining characteristics occur. The Shorr's stain is then applied by dropper, left on for about 1 minute, and the slide is dehydrated by

dipping 3 times into 70% and then 95% alcohol.
It is next blotted and cleared well in xylol.
The slide is then mounted as a permanent preparation.  The entire procedure requires 3
minutes.  Reliance should be placed only on the
picture observed in the thin areas of the slide.

b.  Urinary Gonadotropin (Bioassay)

1)  Significance:  This is a biological test
designed to measure urinary pituitary
gonadotropin concentration.

2)  Method of Assay:  The protein hormone is
precipitated and purified, then it is
injected into immature female mice (white).
Gross enlargement of the uterus occurs if
test is positive.

3)  Normal Values:  Not normally found in urine
before puberty.  Males and females age
20-45 years excrete 6-52 mouse units per
24 hours.  Sexually mature persons between
15 and 20 will also excrete this amount.

4)  Abnormal Values:  Test is not specific for
pituitary gonadotropin, as pregnancy or
chorionepithelioma give high titers.  Serves
to differentiate sexual infantilism or
amenorrhea due to primary end-organ deficiency from that due to pituitary deficiency.
In the former condition FSH may be very high,
whereas in the latter it is low.

5)  Method of Collection:  24 hour urine specimen.
To be stored cold during collection and
frozen as soon as completed.  No preservative
is necessary.

c.  LH and FSH by Radioimmunoassay

Serum LH and FSH may now be measured by radioimmunoassay techniques.  Both tests are performed on 10 ml of clotted blood.

These tests are specific for pituitary,
gonadotropins and are considerably more sensitive
than bioassay methods; n.b., the LH assay does
not distinguish LH from chorionic gonadotropin
(HCG).

Normal values are as follows:

| | FEMALES | | | |
| | FSH in mIU/ml | | LH in mIU/ml | |
| Age | Range | Mean | Range | Mean |
|---|---|---|---|---|
| 2-4 | 3.1- 4.5 | 3.7 | 2.0- 4.0 | 2.8 |
| 5-8 | 3.4- 5.8 | 4.5 | 2.5- 4.0 | 2.6 |
| 9-10 | 3.4- 7.7 | 5.4 | 2.2-12.0 | 4.0 |
| 11-12 | 5.0-12.0 | 7.5 | 2.4-14.0 | 8.7 |
| 13-16 | 3.5-13.3 | 8.0 | 3.8-22.0 | 9.6 |
| 17-18 | 4.4-13.0 | 8.6 | 5.0-29.0 | 15.3 |

| | ADULT FEMALES | | | |
| | FSH in mIU/ml | | LH in mIU/ml | |
| Menstrual Cycle | Range | Mean | Range | Mean |
|---|---|---|---|---|
| Follicular | 4.0-17.2 | 8.3 | 5.0-57.0 | 12.8 |
| Midcycle Peak | 13.7-22.5 | 19.3 | 76.0-90.0 | 83.5 |
| Luteal | 4.0-15.0 | 6.9 | 3.0-41.0 | 11.6 |

| | | MALES | | | |
| | | FSH in mIU/ml | | LH in mIU/ml | |
| Stage* | Age | Range | Mean | Range | Mean |
|---|---|---|---|---|---|
| I | 5-11 | 2.5- 7.0 | 4.5 | 2.5- 5.8 | 3.9 |
| II | 10-13 | 3.0- 9.0 | 5.9 | 4.0-12.0 | 6.8 |
| III | 12-14 | 2.5-14.0 | 8.1 | 6.0-11.0 | 8.5 |
| IV | 12-17 | 3.5-15.0 | 8.5 | 4.0-15.5 | 9.5 |

*Staged according to Tanner, J.M., 1962, Growth at Adolescence, Blackwell and Mott, Ltd., Oxford, pg. 32.

   d. Luteinizing Hormone Releasing Hormone (LH-RH) or Gonadotropin Releasing Hormone (Gn-RH)

   Measures the pituitary LH and FSH reserve and is helpful in the diagnosis of primary (gonadal) versus secondary (pituitary) hypogonadism. The release of LH and FSH in prepubertal children is much less than that in pubertal and past-pubertal children Gn-RH (100µg) is injected intravenously and samples collected for 2 hours. A rise in LH is usually noted by 30 minutes and that for FSH (of much less amplitude) usually noted by 60 minutes.

4. Tests for Human Growth Hormone (hGH)

This hormone may now be measured by a radioimmunoassay technique. However, hGH is not usually found
in the serum unless provocative stimuli are used.
The two standard stimulation tests are: 1) the
response to arginine and 2) the response to insulin
induced hypoglycemia.

Absence of hGH on a screening test is not diagnostic
alone and provocative tests must be performed. Both
tests must be used before an individual is
considered to have no growth hormone response.

a. Screening Tests

   1) Sleep Specimen: A majority of normal sub-
      jects will have a significant release of
      hGH 45-60 minutes after sleep (this applies
      to night time sleep, not naps in infants).
      If a single specimen obtained at this time
      has greater than 5 nanogram/ml, hGH deficiency
      is ruled out.

   2) Exercise Test: Greater than 80% of normals
      will release significant amounts of growth
      hormone following exercise which rules out
      hypopituitarism and obviates a more time-
      consuming tolerance test.

      (a) Procedure:

          (1) Patient must be fasting for at
              least 4 hours.
          (2) After lying still for 30 minutes
              the control sample is drawn.
          (3) The patient then exercises for 20
              minutes consisting of rapid walking
              for 15 minutes followed by rapid
              walking up and down steps for 5
              minutes. It is important that this
              exercise be strenuous. At the
              completion of this time, the second
              sample for growth hormone is drawn.
              After a 20 minute period of lying
              down the final sample is drawn.

      (b) Interpretation: If any one of the three
          samples has greater than 5 nanograms/ml
          of growth hormone, hypopituitarism
          can be excluded.

b.  Arginine-Insulin Tolerance Test

    1)  Necessary Equipment:
        a.  I.V. Volutrole set, 3 way stop clock, arginine solution, 500 ml normal saline and #19 butterfly.
        b.  9 heparinized tubes with suitable tops for use in centrifuge.
        c.  9 tubes with tops for storing plasma.

    2)  Procedure:
        (a)  Start I.V., draw initial sample as control.
        (b)  Arginine is infused over a 30 minute period at a dosage of 0.5 gm/kg/30 min.
        (c)  Bloods drawn as follows:

            0 minutes - control
            15 minutes - Arginine infusing
            30 minutes - Arginine finished
                        (begin normal saline)
            45 minutes -
            60 minutes - Control insulin blood.

        (d)  At 60 minutes of arginine test, inject insulin at dose of 0.075 unit/kg = insulin 0 time.
        (e)  Bloods drawn at 20, 30, 45, 60 minutes after insulin.
        (f)  PATIENT MUST BE OBSERVED DURING ENTIRE TEST FOR SIGNS OF HYPOGLYCEMIA.  A 50% DEXTROSE SOLUTION SHOULD BE KEPT AT THE BEDSIDE.
        (g)  As each specimen is obtained it should be centrifuged and separated.

    3)  Significant Response: >5 nanograms at any time during test.

5.  Steroid Assay Methods (Glucocorticoid Status)

a.  Resting Levels of Urinary 17-Hydroxycorticosteroids (17-OHCS)

    1)  Significance:  The group of steroids measured by this test represents approximately 1/3 of the end products of the metabolism of cortisol (also called hydrocortisone, compound F, 17-hydroxycorticosterone).  Cortisol is the main corticosteroid produced by human adrenals.

2) <u>Technique for Test</u>: A 24 hour urine collection (refrigerate during collection).
No preservative is necessary. The specimens
must be sent to the laboratory <u>immediately</u>
after collection. The 17-OHCS are destroyed
when samples are kept at room temperature
or in a refrigerator but will remain in-
definitely if samples are kept <u>frozen</u>.

3) <u>Normal Values</u>:

| | |
|---|---|
| Adult Males | = 3-9 mg/24 hours |
| Adult Females | = 2-8 mg/24 hours |
| 6 mos-15 yrs | = $3.1 \pm 1.0$ mg/M$^2$/24 hours |

4) <u>Abnormal Values</u>:

The values may be decreased in:
    a) Inanition states: anorexia nervosa.
    b) Pituitary deficiency involving
       adrenocorticotropic hormone.
    c) Addison's disease.
    d) Administration of synthetic, very
       potent corticosteroids such as
       prednisone (Deltasone, Meticorten,
       etc.), triamcinolone (Aristocort,
       Kenacort), dexamethasone (Decadron,
       Deronil, etc.)
    e) Congenital adrenal hyperplasia due
       to 21-hydroxylase deficiency (not
       always).
    f) Liver disease; hypothroidism.
    g) New born period (due to decreased
       glucuronidation, but cortisol
       secretion is not decreased).

The values are increased in:
    a) Cushing's Syndrome.
    b) ACTH, cortisone, cortisol therapy.
    c) Medical and surgical stress (and to
       a lesser degree, emotional stress).
    d) Obesity (not always).
    e) Hyperthyroidism.
    f) Congenital adrenal hyperplasia due
       to 11-hydroxylase deficiency (due
       to 11-deoxycortisol metabolites
       rather than cortisol metabolites).

b. <u>Resting Levels of Urinary 17-Ketosteroids</u>

1) <u>Significance</u>: This group of urinary steroids
represents a part of the end products of
adrenal and testicular androgen metabolism.

2) <u>Method of Assay</u>: The reaction of m-dinitro-benzene in alkaline solution with the group -- $CH_2O$ -- produces a characteris-tic color, which is measured colorimetrically, (Zimmerman reaction).

3) <u>Normal Values</u>:

| | |
|---|---|
| First few weeks | - up to 2 mg/24 hours |
| 1 month-5 years | - 0.5 mg or less/24 hours |
| 6-9 years | - 1-2 mg/24 hours |
| Puberty | - Progressive increase to adult levels |
| Normal adult male | - 7-17 mg/24 hours |
| Normal adult female | - 5-15 mg/24 hours |

4) <u>Abnormal Values</u>: In normal children to 8 years of age and in Addison's Disease, anorexia nervosa, and panhypopituitarism, little or no 17-ketosteroids are found in the urine. Removal of the testes causes a slight decrease. Increases in urinary 17-ketosteroid values may be caused by:
   a) Adrenal hyperplasia.
   b) Virilizing tumor of adrenal cortex.
   c) Cushing's Syndrome (with or without tumor).
   d) Interstitial cell tumor of testes (rare).
   e) Administered hormones such as testos-terone and testosterone propionate (not methyl testosterone), and by ACTH and cortisone.
   f) Alarming stimuli, such as burns, x-ray sickness, etc.

c. <u>Resting Levels of Plasma Corticoids (or Cortisol)</u>

1) <u>Significance</u>: This test measures cortisol, corticosterone, and 11-deoxycortisol (com-pound S). Only the unconjugated steroids are usually measured. But it is also possible to measure those compounds which are conjugated with glucuronic acid.

2) Technique for Test: 2 ml of heparinized blood is required. The cortisol samples must be collected between 8-9 a.m. and sent to the laboratory immediately after collection as plasma must be separated as soon as possible. This is a protein-binding assay. One can separate, if necessary, cortisol from corticosterone and compound S by using an initial paper chromatographic step.

3) Normal values: In addition, radioimmunoassays are available for compound S and cortisol. 12-25 micrograms/100 ml at 8:00 AM and 1-8 micrograms/100 ml late in the evening due to the very marked diurnal variation.

4) Abnormal values: Same as abnormal values for urinary 17-OHCS. However, plasma 17-OHCS are usually normal in anorexia nervosa, liver disease, hypothyroidism, hyperthyroidism, and obesity. Elevated plasma values are found during pregnancy (due to increased concentration of cortisol binding globulin) and during estrogen therapy (particularly women on contraceptive medication). The comparison of 8 AM and 8 PM levels can be useful as screening test for Cushing's.

d. Adrenal Capacity (ACTH Test)

The IM ACTH Test:

1) Significance: Measures the maximal capacity of the adrenal gland to produce cortisol.

2) Technique:

| | |
|---|---|
| Days 1 and 2 | : 24 hours urine collections for control 17-OHCS |
| Days 3,4,5,6 | : Administer IM 40 mg ACTHAR Gel every 12 hours for 4 days (in children: 20 mg/$M^2$ for each injection). Collect 24 hour urine specimins on Days 5 and 6 for urinary 17-OHCS. |

3) Normal Values: Urinary 17-OCHS increase by 5 to 10 times the normal resting 17-OHCS values.

4) Abnormal Values:
   a) A lack of response is pathognomonic of Addison's Disease.
   b) A subnormal response is often found in congenital adrenal hyperplasia.
   c) After cessation of long-term cortisone-like treatment, patients will usually have normal response.
   d) A hyper-response is seen in some cases of Cushing's Syndrome (however, an IV ACTH is more appropriate--see below).

e. The I.V. ACTH Test

   1) Technique: 25 I.U. of ACTH or Synactin (for ACTH usually 1 I.U. = 1 mg; for Synactin 1 I.U. = 0.01 mg) are diluted in 300-500 ml of normal saline or normal glucose and the mixture is given I.V. over a period of 6 hours, starting at 8-9:00 A.M.  Blood samples are taken just prior to the ACTH infusion. If the infusion ends before the end of the 6 hour period, the last blood sample must then be taken at the completion of this infusion.

   2) Normal Values:

      At 6 hours = $40 \pm 6$ µg/100 ml

   3) Abnormal Values: The I.V. ACTH test is of particular interest in Cushing's Syndrome:
      a) A total lack of response is characteristic of an adrenal carcinoma, but a normal response does not exclude a tumor.
      b) A hyper-response is characteristic of bilateral adrenal hyperplasia, but a normal response does not exclude hyper-plasia. In patients whose adrenals have been suppressed for more than one month, the I.V. test is usually not prolonged enough to produce adrenal reactivation.

         An alternative is to use a 24-48 hour continuous infusion ( approximately 80 I.U. per day for adults) and to measure plasma cortisol or urinary steroid metabolites. After the 48 hours infusion there was no overlap in urinary 17-OHCS between normals and patients with either primary or secondary adrenocor-tical insufficiency.

f.  Tests of ACTH Capacity of Pituitary Gland
    (SU-4885, Metyrapone test)

    1)  Significance:  SU-4885 has the property to
        inhibit 11-hydroxylase enzyme in the
        adrenal cortex.  This blocks the normal
        formation of cortisol with decreased blood
        cortisol levels.  If a normally functioning
        pituitary gland is present, a compensatory
        increased secretion of ACTH will result
        in an almost normal secretion of cortisol,
        but also in a large secretion of 11-deoxy-
        precursors of cortisol (compound S).  The
        latter is excreted, like cortisol, as 17-OHCS.

    2)  Technique:

        Days 1 and 2        : No medication.

        Day 3               : Administer orally 500 mg
                              of SU-4885 (Methopyrapone,
                              Ciba) every 4 hours for
                              24 hours (in children:
                              approximately 300 mg/M$^2$
                              every 4 hours for 24 hrs.

        Day 4               : No medication.  Collect
                              24 hour urine collection
                              during the 4 experimental
                              days for urinary 17-OHCS.

    3)  Normal Results:  Urinary 17-OHCS on either
        day 3 or day 4 increased by 2.5 to 6 times
        the normal control 17-OHCS values, and
        should reach a level of 9 mg/M$^2$/24 hrs.
        This test may be modified by using a single
        midnight dose of metyrapone (approximately
        30 mg/kg) and measuring cortisol and compound
        S in the plasma at 8 AM.  A many-fold rise
        in compound S and a precipitous decrease in
        cortisol are found.

        Ref:  Ann. Int. Med. 75:717, 1971.

    4)  Abnormal values:  Little or no response in
        patients with pituitary ACTH deficiency, in
        certain patients with hypothalamic tumors,
        and in subjects who have just stopped
        corticoid therapy (pharmacological
        dosages).  Of course, no response will be
        obtained in patients with primary adrenal
        insufficiency.

5) <u>Insulin induced hypoglycemia</u>: Induce
hypoglycemia with 0.075 to 0.1 units crys-
talline insulin as noted for GH stimulation.
At 0 and 1 hour measure plasma cortisol.
Criteria for normal response are that the
plasma cortisol increment should exceed
5 µg/100 ml and that the maximum level
reached should be greater than 20 µg/100 m

g. <u>Pituitary Suppression Tests</u>

1) <u>Significance</u>: The administration of
dexamethasone, a potent synthetic corticoid,
will suppress ACTH secretion in the normal
subject resulting in decreased endogenous
secretion of cortisol. Since dexamethasone
is not excreted as a 17-OHCS, the values of
urinary 17-OHCS will decrease.

2) <u>Technique</u>:

Days 1 and 2      : No medication

Days 3,4, and 5 : Administer dexamethasone,
1.25 mg/100 lbs of body
weight/day (in 4 divided
doses, every 6 hrs)

Days 6,7, and 8 : Administer dexamethasone,
3.75 mg/100 lbs of body
weight/day (in 4 divided
doses, every 6 hrs)

Collect 24 hour urine collection on experi-
mental days 1,2,4,5,7,8, for urinary 17-
OHCS.

3) <u>Normal Results</u>: By Day 5, the urinary 17-
OHCS have decreased to <2 mg/24 hours.

4) <u>Abnormal Values</u>:
   a) In Cushing's Syndrome from any cause:
      By Day 5, urinary 17-OHCS are
      >2 mg/24 hours.
   b) In Cushing's Syndrome due to bilateral
      adrenal hyperplasia: By Day 8, urinary
      17-OHCS are <2 mg/24 hours, except if
      the hyperplasia is due to an ACTH pro-
      ducing tumor located outside the pitui-
      tary gland (mediastinal, lung, etc.).
   c) In Cushing's Syndrome due to adrenocor-
      tical carcinoma: By Day 8, urinary 17-
      OHCS are >2 mg/24 hours. In certain
      cases of hypothalamic tumor, no suppres-
      sion is obtained.

6. Water Load Test

    a. Method:
       1) N.P.O. after 6 PM.
       2) At 10:30 PM void and discard urine.
       3) Collect and measure subsequent urine to
          7:30 AM.
       4) At 7:30 AM administer 20 ml water/kg PO over
          30 minutes.
       5) Collect and measure urine at 9 AM, 10 AM,
          11 AM, and 12 noon.

    b. Interpretation:
       1) Normal individual excretes 70% of water load.
       2) Normal person excretes greatest volume during
          second hour (10 AM sample).
       3) In the normal, one of the hourly volumes will
          exceed the night volume.

    c. Significance:
       Patients with adrenal cortical insufficiency or
       hypopituitarism are unable to excrete large
       volumes of dilute urine in response to a water
       load.

    NOTE: This test is not valuable in presence of
            diabetes insipidus, renal disease and probably
            liver disease.

            Water load test can be repeated with small
            amounts of cortisol (or ACTH) to determine
            whether patient is hypopituitary, or has
            primary hypoadrenalism.

7. Salt Deprivation Test

Patient is kept on constant low salt diet (9 mEq/day)
for 5 days. Urine and serum electrolytes are
measured.

In normal person after 5 days the serum electrolytes
will be normal and less than 9 mEq/day of sodium
will be excreted.

This test is often carried out along with determination of aldosterone secretion rate. On Day 5,
aldosterone secretion rate should increase 2 to 5
times from the control values of 80 $\pm$ 30 (S.D.)
picogram/24 hours.

8. Prolactin Secretion:

Since prolactin secretion is normally under tonic suppression by prolactin inhibitory factor, disconnection ("functional" or by a space-occupying lesion) causes an increase in the serum concentration. Prolactin concentration also increases after TRH stimulation (see page 79).

Normal Values:

| Female | – 2 to 38 nanograms/ml |
| Male | – 2 to 21 nanograms/ml |
| Prepubertal | – 2 to 21 nanograms/ml |

9. Dehydration Test

Careful dehydration under supervision is the most reliable method to diagnose diabetes insipidus.

a. Method: NPO after test begins and follow urine output and body weight. Measure urine osmolality and creatinine and serum osmolality and Na concentration (see below). Test may be completed by administrating aqueous pitressin 5U, allowing the patient to drink and following urine osmolality.

| Time | Serum Osmolality | Na | Urine Osmolality | Urine Vol | Body Weight |
|------|---|---|---|---|---|
| 8 AM | X | X | X | X | X |
| 9 AM | | | X | X | X |
| 10 AM | X | X | X | X | X |
| 11 AM | | | X | X | X |
| Noon | X | X | X | X | X |

TEST SHOULD BE CONCLUDED IF body weight decreases more than 3%, serum Na >150 mEq/L, urine osmolality >500 mOsM/L, or serum osmolality >300 mOsM/L.

b. Interpretation: After pitressin injection urine osmolality should be greater than serum except in nephrogenic or "metabolic", e.g. hypokalemia, diabetes insipidus.

10. Tests for Pheochromocytoma

    a. Regitine (Phentolamine) Test
       Regitine is an adrenolytic drug used as a
       diagnostic agent in the detection of epinephrine-
       producing tumors of the adrenal or extra-
       adrenal chromaffin tissue.
       1) Method: Do not give a sedative in the
          period before the test.
       2) Dose: 5-10 milligrams in the adult and
          1-5 in the child. It may be given IM or
          IV, but the IV route is preferred.

       The patient should be in the supine position.
       An IV drip should be started with normal saline
       and allowed to drip slowly for 20-30 minutes
       in order to allow the blood pressure to
       stabilize. A blood pressure cuff should be
       attached to the other arm. Three blood pressure
       readings should be obtained after the pressure
       is stabilized, and the last two readings at
       1 minute and 1/2 minute before injection of
       the drug. The drug should be injected over a
       2 minute period slowly. Blood pressure and
       pulse readings should be taken at 1 minute
       intervals for 10-15 minutes after injection. A
       significant blood pressure drop will last 10 min-
       utes or longer. False positive tests may occur.

       3) Side Effects: Symptoms usually occur
          within 1 or 2 minutes and rarely last 3
          minutes. Look for tachycardia, nervousness,
          cold and clammy extremities, hyperpnea,
          mild headache, and precordial distress.

    b. Benzodioxane Test (Benodaine)
       This drug acts in the same was as Regitine,
       but has more side effects.

       Dose: 0.25 milligrams per kg in adults to
       a maximum of 20 milligrams. In children the
       dose must be calculated from a basal metabo-
       lism nomogram and is 10 milligrams/$M^2$.

    c. Catecholamines in the Urine
       This is a more specific test for epinephrine
       and norepinephrine secreting tumors. It should
       be relied on whenever time permits its usage.
       A 24 hour sample of urine is sent to the
       chemistry laboratory. Sample should be pro-
       tected from light and should have 8 ml of
       concentrated HCl added during collection.
       If possible urine should be obtained during
       a paroxysm of hypertension.

       Normal: Less than 100 micrograms/24 hours.

d. Vanillyl Mandelic Acid (VMA)
3-Methoxy-4-Hydroxy Mandelic Acid:  This
metabolite of adrenalin and noradrenalin may
be found elevated in cases of pheochromocytoma
or neuroblastoma which do not show an elevated
catecholamine urine level.

There is a paper chromatographic and a color-
imeter method of determination.

No fruits, tea, coffee, or vanilla-containing
foods for at least 24 hours.

Collect 24 hour urine, acidified with 15 cc
of concentrated HCl.

Normal:  3-9 µg/mg creatinine.

Ref:  Arch. Dis. Child. 39:168, 1964.

e. Homovanillic Acid (HVA)
This metabolite is a common end product of
DOPA and DOPAMINE, precursors of the catechol-
amines.  HVA excretion is independent of dietary
factors.  Patients with neuroblastoma show a
marked increase in HVA excretion, while those
with pheochromocytoma excrete normal amounts
of HVA.  The DOPA and DOPAMINE assay may be
substituted for this determination of HVA.

As with VMA a 24 hour urine is collected in
a dark bottle, with 5-10 ml of 6 N HCl added.

Normal:  50 µg/mg creatinine.

Ref:  Arch. Dis. Child. 39:168, 1964.

11. Tests of Parathyroid Function

a. Serum Calcium and Phosphate Levels:  These
concentrations are very helpful for the
diagnosis of hypo- and hyperparathyroidism,
especially when combined with a measurement
of the parathyroid hormone (PTH) concentration.

b. Urinary Cyclic Adenosine 3', 5' - Monophosphate
(3', 5' AMP):  Urinary excretion of 3', 5' -
AMP is measured basally and after a 15 minute
infusion of parathyroid hormone (100 to 300
units). PTH causes a marked increase in the
excretion of 3', 5' - AMP except in patients
with pseudohypoparathyroidism and is consequently
diagnostic for this familial disease.

Ref:  J. Clin. Invest. 48:1832, 1969.
J. Clin. Endocrinol. Metabol. 37:476, 1973.

c. Parathyroid Hormone (PTH) Concentration: At present this test is not routinely performed; however, when available, increased concentrations of PTH in the presence of hypercalcemia is diagnostic of hyperparathyroidism. PTH concentration is also increased in pseudo-hypoparathyroidism.

12. Bone Age:

a. Wrist and Hand: Read by the method of Greulich and Pyle.

   Ref: Radiographic Atlas of Skeletal Development of the Hand and Wrist, 2nd ed. Stanford, Calif., Stanford University press, 1959.

b. Knee: Read by method of Pyle and Hoerr.

   Ref: Radiographic Atlas of Skeletal Development of the Knee, Springfield, Ill., Charles C. Thomas, 1969.

c. By special request hemiskeleton views may be taken to be read by the method of Wilkins.

   Ref: Diagnosis and Treatment of Endocrine Disorders in Childhood and Adolescence, 3rd ed. Springfield, Ill., Charles C. Thomas, 1965.

## DIAGNOSTIC METHODS FOR HORMONAL DISORDERS

| Hormone | Clinical Tests | Assays | Chemical Determination Urine | Chemical Determination Serum |
|---|---|---|---|---|
| **Pituitary Hormones** | | | | |
| hGH | Exercise<br>Arginine tolerance test<br>Insulin tolerance test<br>L-DOPA test | *RIA-serum | | |
| TSH | Response of 131I uptake to TSH<br>TRH infusion | RIA-serum | | |
| ACTH | Dexamethasone suppression of 17-OHCS<br>Metyrapone (SU-4855) effect on 17-OHCS | Bioassay | | Compound S,F |
| FSH | Gonadotropin hormone | RIA-serum | | |
| LH | Releasing hormone | RIA-serum | | |
| HCG | | RIA-serum | | |
| Prolactin | TRH infusion | RIA-serum | | |
| Total Gonadotropins | | Bioassay of urine-uterine weight in immature mouse | | |

*RIA = radioimmunossay

DIAGNOSTIC METHODS FOR HORMONAL DISORDERS (continued)

| Hormone | Clinical Tests | Assays | Chemical Determination Urine | Chemical Determination Serum |
|---|---|---|---|---|
| Thyroid Hormones | 131 I Uptake<br>T3 suppression test | *RIA for T4, T3 | | T4 by column<br>T4(C)<br>T4-Murphy<br>Patte T4(D)<br>Free T4<br>TBG |
| Adrenal Medullary Hormones | | | | |
| Epinephrine and/or Norepinephrine | Histamine test<br>Regitine test | Bioassay for epinephrine | Epine-phrine & Norepine-phrine VMA, HVA | Epinephrine & norepine-phrine |
| Adrenocortical Hormones | | | | |
| Aldosterone | Serum Na, K, CO2, Cl<br>Sweat and saliva Na/K<br>Response to Na deprivation<br>Response to aldactone<br>Aldosterone secretory rate | Na retention in adrenalectomized rats | Aldoster-one | Aldosterone |

*RIA = radioimmunoassay

DIAGNOSTIC METHODS FOR HORMONAL DISORDERS (continued)

| Hormone | Clinical Tests | Assays | Chemical Determination | |
|---|---|---|---|---|
| | | | Urine | Serum |
| Cortisol | "Water load test"<br>Effect of ACTH on 17-OHCS<br>Effect of dexamethasone on 17-OHCS<br>Effect of SU-4885 on 17-OHCS<br>Cortisol secretory rate | Bioassay | 17-OHCS<br>17-Keto-genic | 17-OHCS<br>Cortisol |
| Adrenal Androgens | Suppression by dexa-methasone of 17-KS | Bioassay | 17-KS<br>11-oxy-17-KS | 17-KS |
| Testicular Hormones | Lack of suppression of 17-KS by dexamethasone | Bioassay | 17-KS<br>Testos-terone | 17-KS |
| Ovarian Hormones | | | | |
| Estrogens | Vaginal smear or biopsy<br>Endometrial biopsy | | Estrogen | Estrogen |
| Progesterone | Basal temperature curve<br>Endometrial biopsy<br>Vaginal smear | Bioassay | Pregnane-diol | |

# P S Y C H O L O G I C A L

## T E S T I N G

The following screening tests are aimed at providing the pediatrician with appropriate tools with which to determine whether or not a child should be referred for more exhaustive examination regarding the possibility of mental retardation.

Brief screening tools always bring with them a certain amount of error. The child with normal learning capacity may not be able to respond very well to a specific tool because it happens to touch an ability area that he is not particularly strong in. Hence, a child may be falsely identified as retarded. A child may also be able to draw a human figure quite well but at the same time he may have a serious language handicap producing a specific learning disability. To use the brief screening tool to claim that there are no cognitive deficits to be concerned about is an example of improper use of a psychological tool.

The pediatrician therefore has to make a reasonable decision based on his impression of the child and on the presenting complaint. For example, a complaint that the child is doing very poorly in school automatically requires the intervention of a professional psychologist. The child may look normal on a screening test but may still be an example of a specific learning disability. He may appear retarded on your screening tests, but, again, may be of normal intellectual ability while demonstrating a specific handicap.

The following tests are included because of their ease of administration and demonstrated reliability.

### GOODENOUGH-HARRIS DRAW-A-PERSON TEST

1. Procedure: The child is supplied with a pencil (preferably a No. 2 with eraser) and a sheet of blank paper and instructed to "Draw a person", "Draw the best person you can". No additional directions are necessary. Encouragement may be supplied if necessary. Under no condition should the examiner suggest that the child's production needs to be supplemented or changed in any way; the only exception being the drawing of the stick figure. In this case the examiner is permitted to encourage the child to "draw a whole person."

2. Scoring: The child receives one point for each detail present according to the following scoring guides:

## Drawing of a Man

1. Head present
2. Neck present
3. Neck , two dimensions
4. Eyes present
5. Eye detail: brow or lashes
6. Eye detail: pupil
7. Nose present
8. Nose, two dimensions (not round ball)
9. Mouth present
10. Lips, two dimensions
11. Both nose and lips in two dimensions
12. Both chin and forehead shown
13. Bridge of nose (straight to eyes; narrower than base)
14. Hair I (any scribble)
15. Hair II (more detail)
16. Ears present
17. Fingers present
18. Correct number of fingers shown
19. Opposition of thumb shown (must include fingers)
20. Hands present
21. Arms present
22. Arms at side or engaged in activity
23. Feet: any indication
24. Attachment of arms and legs I (to trunk anywhere)
25. Attachment of arms and legs II (at correct point of trunk)
26. Trunk present
27. Trunk in proportion, two dimensions (length greater than breadth)
28. Clothing I (anything)
29. Clothing II (2 articles of clothing)

## Drawing of a Woman

1. Head present
2. Neck present
3. Neck, two dimensions
4. Eyes present
5. Eye detail: brow or lashes
6. Eye detail: pupil
7. Nose present (not round ball)
8. Nose, two dimensions
9. Bridge of nose (straight to eyes, narrower than base)
10. Nostrils shown
11. Mouth present
12. Lips, two dimensions
13. Both nose and lips in two dimensions
14. Both chin and forehead shown
15. Hair I (any scribble)
16. Hair II (more detail)
17. Necklace or earrings
18. Arms present
19. Fingers present
20. Correct number of fingers shown
21. Opposition of thumb shown (must include fingers)
22. Hands present
23. Legs present
24. Feet (any indication)
25. Shoe "feminine" (any attempt such as high heels, open toe, strap)
26. Attachment of arms and legs I (to trunk anywhere)
27. Attachment of arms and legs II (to trunk at correct point)
28. Clothing indicated (any)
29. Sleeve
30. Neckline (any indication)
31. Trunk present
32. Trunk in proportion, two dimensions (length greater than breadth)

3. <u>Norms</u>: minimum score for child to be within one standard deviation of age - appropriate mean.

| Age | Drawing of Man | | Drawing of Woman | |
|-----|----------------|-----------|------------------|-----------|
|     | by boys | by girls | by boys | by girls |
| 3 | 4 | 5 | 4 | 6 |
| 4 | 7 | 7 | 7 | 8 |
| 5 | 11 | 12 | 11 | 14 |
| 6 | 13 | 14 | 13 | 16 |
| 7 | 16 | 17 | 16 | 19 |
| 8 | 18 | 20 | 20 | 23 |

## DEVELOPMENTAL ASSESSMENT

On the following pages there are two additional, but different, tests for assessing development. One is the well-known Denver Developmental Screening Test which objectively assesses a child's performance of certain maneuvers and tasks. The other is an evaluation utilizing an interview technique by asking parents a list of questions regarding milestones and achievements which most will remember. This has been very successful in its use at the John F. Kennedy Institute for the Habilitation of Handicapped Children at Johns Hopkins. Both have their own advantages and must be adapted to the individual situation depending on the child, parents, and examiner.

## DEVELOPMENTAL ASSESSMENT BY INTERVIEW

| Age | Gross Motor | Fine Motor | Language | Social |
|-----|-------------|------------|----------|--------|
| 3 mo. | A. Does he support himself on forearms when lying? | A. Are his hands usually open at rest? | A. Does he laugh or make happy noises? | A. Does he smile at you? |
| | B. Does he hold his head up steadily while on his stomach? | B. Does he pull at his clothing? | B. Does he turn his head to sounds? | B. Does he reach for familiar people or objects? |
| 6 mo. | A. Does he lift his head when lying on his back? | A. Does he transfer a toy from one hand to the other? | A. Does he "babble", repeat sounds together (i.e., mum-mum-mum)? | A. Does he stretch his arms out to be picked up? |
| | B. Does he roll from back to front? | B. Does he pick up small objects? | B. Is he frightened by angry noise? | B. Does he show his likes and dislikes? |
| 9 mo. | A. Does he sit for long periods without support? | A. Does he pick up objects with his thumb and one finger? | A. Does he understand "no-no", "bye-bye"? | A. Does he hold his own bottle? |
| | B. Does he pull up on furniture? | B. Does he finger-feed any foods? | B. Will he imitate any sounds or words if you make them first? | B. Does he play any nursery games ("peek-a-boo", "bye-bye")? |

DEVELOPMENTAL ASSESSMENT BY INTERVIEW (continued)

| Age | Gross Motor | Fine Motor | Language | Social |
|---|---|---|---|---|
| 12 mo. | A. Is he walking (alone or with hand held)? | A. Does he throw toys (objects)? | A. Does he have at least one meaning-ful word other than "mama", "dada"? | A. Does he cooperate in dressing? |
| | B. Does he pivot when sitting? | B. Does he give you toys (let go) easily? | B. Does he shake his head for "no"? | B. Does he come when you call him? |
| 18 mo. | A. Does he walk up-stairs with help? | A. Does he turn book pages (2 or 3 at a time)? | A. Does he have at least 6 real words besides his "jar-gon"? | A. Does he copy you in routine tasks (sweeping, dusting, etc.)? |
| | B. Can he throw a toy while stand-ing without falling? | B. Does he fill spoon and feed self? | B. Does he point at at what he wants? | B. Does he play in the company of other children? |
| 2 yr. | A. Does he run well without falling? | A. Does he turn book pages one at a time? | A. Does he talk in short (2-3 word) sentences? | A. Does he ask to be taken to the toilet? |
| | B. Does he walk up and down stairs alone? | B. Does he remove his own shoes, pants? | B. Does he use pro-nouns ("me", "you", "mine")? | B. Does he play in company of other children? |
| 2½ yr. | A. Does he jump, getting both feet off the floor? | A. Does he unbutton any buttons? | A. Does he use plu-rals or past tense? | A. Does he tell his first and last name if asked? |
| | B. Does he throw a ball overhand? | B. Does he hold a pencil or crayon adult fashion? | B. Does he use the word "I" correctly most of the time? | B. Does he get him-self a drink with-out help? |

DEVELOPMENTAL ASSESSMENT BY INTERVIEW (continued)

| Age | Gross Motor | Fine Motor | Language | Social |
|---|---|---|---|---|
| 3 yr. | A. Does he pedal a tricycle? | A. Does he dry his hands (if reminded)? | A. Does he tell little stories about his experiences? | A. Does he share his toys? |
| | B. Does he alternate feet (one stair per step) going upstairs? | B. Does he dress and undress fully including front buttons? | B. Does he know his sex? | B. Does he play well with another child? Take turns? |
| 4 yr. | A. Does he attempt to hop or skip? | A. Does he button clothes fully? | A. Does he say a song or a poem from memory? | A. Does he tell "tall tales" or "show off"? |
| | B. Does he alternate feet going downstairs? | B. Does he catch a ball? | B. Does he know all his colors? | B. Does he play cooperatively with a small group of children? |
| 5 yr. | A. Does he skip, alternating feet? | A. Does he tie his own shoes? | A. Can he print his first name? | A. Is he a "mother's helper", likes to do things for you? |
| | B. Does he jump rope or jump over low obstacles? | B. Does he spread with a knife? | B. Does he ever ask what a word means? | B. Does he play competitive games and abide by the rules? |

Adapted from Capute and Biehl, Ped Clin N.A. 20:3, 1960

106

1. Try to get child to smile by smiling, talking or waving to him. Do not touch him.
2. When child is playing with toy, pull it away from him. Pass if he resists.
3. Child does not have to be able to tie shoes or button in the back.
4. Move yarn slowly in an arc from one side to the other, about 6" above child's face.
   Pass if eyes follow 90° to midline. (Past midline; 180°)
5. Pass if child grasps rattle when it is touched to the backs or tips of fingers.
6. Pass if child continues to look where yarn disappeared or tries to see where it went. Yarn
   should be dropped quickly from sight from tester's hand without arm movement.
7. Pass if child picks up raisin with any part of thumb and a finger.
8. Pass if child picks up raisin with the ends of thumb and index finger using an over hand approach.

9. Pass any en-
   closed form.
   Fail continuous
   round motions.

10. Which line is longer?
    (Not bigger.) Turn
    paper upside down and
    repeat. (3/3 or 5/6)

11. Pass any
    crossing
    lines.

12. Have child copy
    first. If failed,
    demonstrate

13. When scoring, each pair (2 arms, 2 legs, etc.) counts as one part.
14. Point to picture and have child name it. (No credit is given for sounds only.)

105

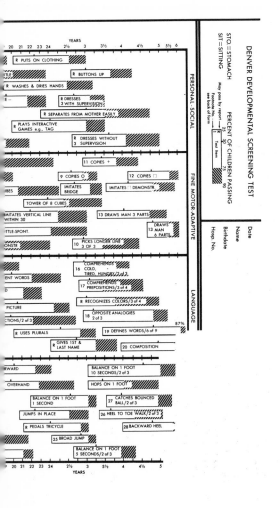

DENVER DEVELOPMENTAL SCREENING TEST

STO.=STOMACH
SIT.=SITTING

PERCENT OF CHILDREN PASSING

May pass by report
Footnote No. —
see back of form

Test Item

Date
Name
Birthdate
Hosp. No.

**PERSONAL-SOCIAL**

R PUTS ON CLOTHING
R BUTTONS UP
R WASHES & DRIES HANDS
R DRESSES 3 WITH SUPERVISION
R SEPARATES FROM MOTHER EASILY
R PLAYS INTERACTIVE GAMES e.g., TAG
R DRESSES WITHOUT 3 SUPERVISION

**FINE MOTOR-ADAPTIVE**

11 COPIES +
9 COPIES O          12 COPIES □
IMITATES BRIDGE     IMITATES □ DEMONSTR.
TOWER OF 8 CUBES
IMITATES VERTICAL LINE WITHIN 30    13 DRAWS MAN 3 PARTS
DRAWS 13 MAN 6 PARTS
10 PICKS LONGER LINE 3 OF 3

**LANGUAGE**

16 COMPREHENDS COLD, TIRED, HUNGRY/2 of 3
17 COMPREHENDS PREPOSITIONS/3 of 4
R RECOGNIZES COLORS/3 of 3
18 OPPOSITE ANALOGIES 2 of 3
R USES PLURALS
R GIVES 1ST & LAST NAME
19 DEFINES WORDS/6 of 9
20 COMPOSITION

87%

BALANCE ON 1 FOOT 10 SECONDS/2 of 3
HOPS ON 1 FOOT
BALANCE ON 1 FOOT 1 SECOND
27 CATCHES BOUNCED BALL/2 of 3
JUMPS IN PLACE
26 HEEL TO TOE WALK/2 of 3
R PEDALS TRICYCLE
28 BACKWARD HEEL
25 BROAD JUMP
BALANCE ON 1 FOOT 5 SECONDS/2 of 3

YEARS
20 21 22 23 24   2½   3   3½   4   4½   5

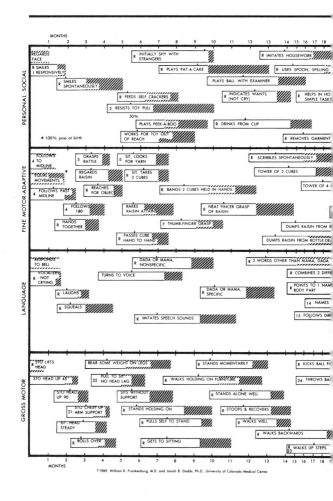

Denver Developmental Screening Test

MONTHS
1  2  3  4  5  6  7  8  9  10  11  12  13  14  15  16  17  18

**PERSONAL-SOCIAL**

REGARDS FACE
R SMILES RESPONSIVELY
R SMILES SPONTANEOUSLY
R FEEDS SELF CRACKERS
2 RESISTS TOY PULL
PLAYS PEEK-A-BOO
WORKS FOR TOY OUT OF REACH
R INITIALLY SHY WITH STRANGERS
R PLAYS PAT-A-CAKE
PLAYS BALL WITH EXAMINER
R INDICATES WANTS (NOT CRY)
R DRINKS FROM CUP
R IMITATES HOUSEWORK
R USES SPOON, SPILLING
HELPS IN HOUSE SIMPLE TASKS
R REMOVES GARMENT

50%

★ 100% poss at birth

**FINE MOTOR-ADAPTIVE**

FOLLOWS TO MIDLINE
EQUAL MOVEMENTS
FOLLOWS PAST MIDLINE
R HANDS TOGETHER
R FOLLOWS 180
5 GRASPS RATTLE
REGARDS RAISIN
R REACHES FOR OBJECT
RAKES RAISIN ATTAIN
PASSES CUBE HAND TO HAND
6 SIT, LOOKS FOR YARN
SIT, TAKES 2 CUBES
R BANGS 2 CUBES HELD IN HANDS
7 THUMB-FINGER GRASP
8 NEAT PINCER GRASP OF RAISIN
R SCRIBBLES SPONTANEOUSLY
TOWER OF 2 CUBES
TOWER OF 4
DUMPS RAISIN FROM B
DUMPS RAISIN FROM BOTTLE-DE

**LANGUAGE**

RESPONDS TO BELL
VOCALIZES R - NOT CRYING
R LAUGHS
R SQUEALS
TURNS TO VOICE
R IMITATES SPEECH SOUNDS
DADA OR MAMA, NONSPECIFIC
DADA OR MAMA, SPECIFIC
R 3 WORDS OTHER THAN MAMA, DADA
R COMBINES 2 DIFF
R POINTS TO 1 NAM BODY PART
14 NAMES
15 FOLLOWS DIR

**GROSS MOTOR**

STO LIFTS HEAD
STO HEAD UP 45°
STO HEAD UP 90°
STO CHEST UP 21 ARM SUPPORT
SIT - HEAD STEADY
R ROLLS OVER
BEAR SOME WEIGHT ON LEGS
PULL TO SIT 22 NO HEAD LAG
SITS WITHOUT SUPPORT
R STANDS HOLDING ON
R PULLS SELF TO STAND
R GETS TO SITTING
R STANDS MOMENTARILY
R WALKS HOLDING ON FURNITURE
R STANDS ALONE WELL
R STOOPS & RECOVERS
R WALKS WELL
R WALKS BACKWARDS
R KICKS BALL F
24 THROWS BA
R WALKS UP STEPS 23

1  2  3  4  5  6  7  8  9  10  11  12  13  14  15  16  17  18
MONTHS

©1969, William K. Frankenburg, M.D. and Josiah B. Dodds, Ph.D., University of Colorado Medical Center.

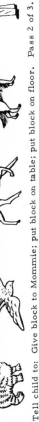

15. Tell child to: Give block to Mommie; put block on table; put block on floor.   Pass 2 of 3.
    (Do not help child by pointing, moving head or eyes.)

16. Ask child: What do you do when you are cold? ..hungry? ..tired?   Pass 2 of 3.

17. Tell child to: Put block on table; under table; in front of chair, behind chair.
    Pass 3 of 4.   (Do not help child by pointing, moving head or eyes.)

18. Ask child: If fire is hot, ice is ?; Mother is a woman, Dad is a ?; a horse is big, a
    mouse is ?.   Pass 2 of 3.

19. Ask child: What is a ball? ..lake? ..desk? ..house? ..banana? ..curtain? ..ceiling?
    ..hedge? ..pavement?   Pass if defined in terms of use, shape, what it is made of or general
    category (such as banana is fruit, not just yellow).   Pass 6 of 9.

20. Ask child: What is a spoon made of? ..a shoe made of? ..a door made of?   (No other objects
    may be substituted.)   Pass 3 of 3.

21. When placed on stomach, child lifts chest off table with support of forearms and/or hands.

22. When child is on back, grasp his hands and pull him to sitting.   Pass if head does not hang back.

23. Child may use wall or rail only, not person.   May not crawl.

24. Child must throw ball overhand 3 feet to within arm's reach of tester.

25. Child must perform standing broad jump over width of test sheet.   (8-1/2 inches)

26. Tell child to walk forward,   heel within 1 inch of toe.
    Tester may demonstrate.   Child must walk 4 consecutive steps, 2 out of 3 trials.

27. Bounce ball to child who should stand 3 feet away from tester.   Child must catch ball with
    hands, not arms, 2 out of 3 trials.

28. Tell child to walk backward,   toe within 1 inch of heel.
    Tester may demonstrate.   Child must walk 4 consecutive steps, 2 out of 3 trials.

DATE AND BEHAVIORAL OBSERVATIONS (how child feels at time of test, relation to tester, attention
span, verbal behavior, self-confidence, etc.):

S K I N   T E S T S

1. Cat Scratch Disease Skin Test

   Antigen prepared from involved lymph nodes of
   infected human.  Dose:  0.1 ml of antigen ID.
   Interpretation:  Read at 24 hours.  Positive area
   of erythema and induration 2-4 cm in diameter with
   central 6-8 papule.

2. Chancroid Skin Test

   Saline suspension of killed Hemophilus ducreyi
   organisms.  Dose:  0.05 ml ID.  Interpretation:
   Read at 48 hours.  Positive reaction consists of
   induration over 2 cm in diameter, remains positive
   after recovery and therefore does not distinguish
   past from present infection.

3. Coccidioidin Skin Test

   1:100 dilution of filtrate of a selected strain
   of Coccidioides immitis.  Dose:  Dilute 1:100 to
   1:1000 and inject 0.1 ml of latter ID.  Read at
   48 hours.  If negative, repeat with 1:100.
   Interpretation:  Read at 48 hours.  Induration over
   1.5 cm in diameter is positive.  Positive reaction
   usually obtained 2-4 weeks post infection, remain
   positive for years.

4. Echinococcus Skin Test

   Antigen obtained from dog tapeworm or from hyda-
   tid fluid.  Dose:  0.25 ml ID with nearby control
   saline injection.  Interpretation:  Read at 1/2
   hour and 24 hours.  Initial blanching of test
   area usually increases and may show pseudopods.
   Positive 1/2 hour reaction has wheal at least 2.4
   cm in one diameter, or 2.2 cm in both diameters.
   Positive 24 hour reaction has infiltration and edema
   at least 4 cm in diameter.  Indicates present or
   past infection, remains positive for life.

5. Histoplasmin Skin Test

   Culture filtrate of Hist. capsulatum.  Dose: 0.1
   ml of 1:100 dilution ID.  Interpretation:  Read
   at 48 and 72 hours.  Positive if at either reading
   induration is more than 0.5 cm in diameter.  Cross
   reaction may occur with other fungi (B. dermatiti-
   dis, C. immitis, or C. albicans).  Skin testing may
   stimulate a falsely positive complement fixation
   test for histoplasmosis.

6. Lymphogranuloma Venereum Skin Test (Frei Test)

Antigen prepared from chick-embryo grown virus.
Dose: 0.1 ml ID and control. Interpretation:
Read at 48 and 72 hours. Positive is reddish
papule 6 mm or more in diameter surrounded by
faint erythematous area. Use control to rule out
sensitivity to chick protein. Reaction remains
positive after infection for many years. Cross
reaction may occur with psittacosis group of
viruses.

7. Moloney Test for Diphtheria Toxoid Sensitivity
(Modified)

1:100 dilution of fluid toxoid to determine degree
of sensitivity to diphtheria toxoid prior to its
use in active immunization of children over 10
years and adults. Dose: 0.1 ml ID. Interpretation: Read at 48 hours. Reaction positive if
erythema more than 1.0 cm in diameter. Positive
test calls for most cautious use of diphtheria
toxoid.

8. Mumps Skin Test

Killed virus suspension prepared from extra-
embryonic fluid of infected chick embryos to determine susceptibility to mumps during or after
adolescence. Dose: 0.1 ml ID. Interpretation:
Read at 24 and 36 hours. Immunity is indicated
by induration and erythema 1.5 cm or more in
diameter. There are considerable false negatives
and a mumps complement fixation titer is a
more reliable determination.

Ref: J. Pediat. 62:604, 1963.

9. Sarcoid Skin Test (Kveim)

Ground sarcoid lymph nodes tested for sterility
and preserved with phenol. Dose: 0.1-0.2 ml ID.
Interpretation: Red-purple papule appears in 7-14
days, grows slowly for 4-6 weeks. When papule
maximal in size (3-8 mm) biopsy of papule in positive test shows epithelioid and giant cells
surrounded by inflammatory cells. Reports vary
concerning efficiency (64-94%) in diagnosis.

10. <u>Shick Test</u>

Sterile solution of toxic growth products of C. diphtheriae. Dose: 0.1 ml (1/50 M.L.D. of toxin) ID. Interpretation: Read in 3-4 days. Positive reaction (non-immune) consists of circumscribed redness and infiltration 1-2 cm in diameter.

11. <u>Toxoplasma Skin Test</u>

Extract of killed organisms. Dose: 0.1 ml (1:500) ID. Interpretation: Read at 24 and 48 hours. Positive result induration 0.5 cm in diameter. False positive results may occur.

12. <u>Trichinella Skin Test</u>

Extract of dried, ground trichinellae. Dose: 0.01-0.02 ml ID with saline control. Interpretation: Observe for 24 hours. Positive reaction is of immediate type, usually within 15-20 minutes after injection, rarely delayed to 24 hours, and consists of induration of 1-3 cm or of erythema of 1-5 cm. Control rarely shows induration more than 0.3 cm and erythema more than 0.5 cm. Tests usually not positive until second week of infection. Normals may have positive reactions from previous unrecognized trichinosis or crossreacting parasites, such as trichuris trichiura.

13. <u>Tuberculin Tests</u>

| International Units | Old Tuberculin Dose | Dilution | PPD Strength |
|---|---|---|---|
| 1 | 0.01 mg | 1:10,000 | First |
| 5 | 0.05 | 1:2,000 | Intermed = Tine |
| 10 | 0.10 | 1:1,000 | = Patch (Vollmer) |
| 100 | 1.00 | 1:100 | Second |

Methods:
a. Intradermal: Inject 0.1 ml of test material. Record mm of induration after 2-3 days. Interpretation: <5 mm induration is negative; 5 mm to 9 mm is consistent with M. Tuberculosis, atypical mycobacteria, or previous BCG; 10 mm or greater is almost always only M. tuberculosis.

b.  Tine: Press disc firmly into the skin of the
    alcohol washed and dried forearm, using enough
    pressure to leave 4 visible puncture sites.
    Measure induration after 2-3 days. Interpre-
    tation: 2 mm induration around any one point
    is equivalent to 5 mm induration with 0.05 mg OT.
    Positive reactions tend to coalesce.
c.  Patch Test: Not used because of high incidence
    of false negative reactions.

NOTES:
1.  Subcutaneous injection or not injecting
    exactly 0.1 ml makes quantitation invalid.
2.  5 Tuberculin Units used for routine
    screening: 1 TU may give false negatives,
    and 100-250 TU may give false positives and
    severe reactions.

14. Candida and Trichophyton Skin Tests

A dose of 0.1 ml of a stock solution (1:1000) is
injected ID and read at 24 and 48 hours. Erythema
or induration of 5 mm or more is evidence of an
ability to mount a delayed hypersensitivity reaction.

PREPARATIONS FOR X-RAY EXAMINATIONS

N.B.   In order to avoid inadvertent irradiation of a
fetus or embryo, NO DIAGNOSTIC ROENTGENOGRAMS
SHOULD BE MADE OF THE ABDOMEN, PELVIS, HIPS OR
THIGHS (including upper gastrointestinal series,
barium enema, excretory urogram) OF GIRLS AGE 12
OR OLDER EXCEPT DURING THE FIRST TEN DAYS OF THE
MENSTRUAL CYCLE, COUNTING FROM THE FIRST DAY OF
THE PERIOD, and all other roentgenographic examinations should be kept to a minimum with the lower
abdomen and pelvis shielded.  This policy does not
apply to women on contraceptive pills or having
an intra-uterine device.

1.   Psychological Preparation

The child should be prepared for the examination,
either by hospital personnel or his parents.  If
the child is an outpatient, the parents should be
told enough about the examination so that they under-
stand what the child will experience.

2.   Bisacodyl (Dulcolax)

Tablets should not be taken within 1 hour of
antacids or milk.  They must not be chewed or
crushed, but rather swallowed whole.  Use suppositories unless you are certain the child can swallow
the tablets whole.  Dose: Below 40 kg: 1 tablet
h.s.; above 40 kg: 2 tablets h.s.

Suppositories may be used at any age.  If the first
suppository does not produce a good bowel movement
within 45 minutes, administer a second suppository.

Contraindications: Acute surgical abdomen, acute
ulcerative colitis.

3.   Upper Gastrointestinal Series

(A small bowel follow-through is part of each upper
gastrointestinal series, except when there is severe
gastric or duodenal obstruction.)

a.   Patient less than 18 months old:
     1.   Nothing by mouth for 3 hours before the
          examination and until completed.
     2.   Bisacodyl suppository:  one 90 minutes
          before the examination, and repeat in 45
          minutes if the patient does not have a
          large bowel movement.
b.   Patient 19 months or older:
     1.   Bisacodyl pill(s) or suppository h.s.
          (see 2).

    2. Nothing by mouth for 4 to 6 hours (depending on size) before the examination and until completed.

    3. Bisacodyl suppository: one 90 minutes before the examination and repeat in 45 minutes if the patient does not have a large bowel movement.

4. Air Contrast Barium Enema

    a. Patients less than 3 years old:
   Arrangements must be made with the pediatric radiologist for this special examination and the correct preparation.

    b. Patients 3 years of age and older:
   1. Clear liquid diet for 48 hours before examination. No milk or dairy products.
   2. 36 hours before examination: bisacodyl pill(s) or suppository (see 2).
   3. 24 hours before examination: bisacodyl suppository (see 2).
   4. 12 hours before the examination: saline enemas until clear.
   5. N.P.O. for 3 hours before the examination.

5. Regular Barium Enema

(Omit steps b and d when evaluation is for possible Hirschsprung's disease, ulcerative colitis, or acute surgical abdomen.)

    a. Clear liquid diet for 24 hours before the examination. No milk or dairy products, except that infants may have regular formula.

    b. Bisacodyl pill(s) or suppository h.s. (see 2).

    c. N.P.O. for 4 hours (infants, 3 hours) before the examination and until completed.

    d. Bisacodyl suppository: one 90 minutes before the examination, and repeat in 45 minutes if the patient does not have a large bowel movement

6. Excretory Urogram (IVP)

    a. The patient should be normally hydrated but have an empty stomach. With the doses of contrast material recommended, dehydration prior to the procedure is contraindicated at all ages, and especially dangerous in infants or if there is uremia.

    b. An infant's feedings should be arranged so that the examination is started at the time of the next feeding; the feeding may be given as soon as the injection has been completed. Children should be N.P.O. for 4 to 6 hours (depending on size) before the examination.

c. A carbonated beverage is frequently given during the examination. Be certain to indicate on the requisition if this sugar containing beverage is contraindicated.

d. Bisacodyl suppository: one 90 minutes before the examination, and repeat in 45 minutes if patient does not have a large bowel movement.

e. Have patient void just before examination.

f. Dose: Renografin-60

| | |
|---|---|
| 0 - 2.5 kg. | By consultation with the Pediatric Radiology staff |
| 2.5 - 6 kg. | 3 ml/kg. |
| 7 - 10 kg. | 20 ml |
| 11 - 25 kg. | 2 ml/kg. |
| above 25 kg. | 50 ml (maximum dose) |

7. Cystourethrogram

a. N.P.O. for three hours before the examination.

8. Herniogram (Positive Contrast Peritoneal Study)

a. Requires consent sheet to be signed by parent or guardian.

b. N.P.O. for three hours before the examination.

c. Contraindications:
   1. Hypersensitivity to contrast material.
   2. Urinary retention.
   3. Peritonitis.
   4. Distended bowel (mechanical obstruction, paralytic ileus, gastroenteritis, etc.).
   5. Ventriculo-peritoneal shunt for hydro-cephalus.
   6. Bleeding tendency.
   7. Abdominal wall infection.

9. Pelvic Pneumography

a. Requires consent sheet to be signed by parent or guardian.

b. Same preparation as for regular barium enema.

10. Cholecystogram

a. The diet should contain fat the day before the examination. On the evening of the examination, however, give a light meal that avoids all fat, including eggs, milk and other dairy products.

b. Iopanoic acid (Telepaque) 0.5 gm (one tablet) for each 10 kg of body weight, not to exceed 3.0 gm (6 tablets). Starting after dinner,

give 1 tablet each 15 minutes with water.  The
tablets may be crushed and administered in food.

c.  N.P.O., except ordinary amounts of water,
following the iopanoic acid until the examination.  Infants should have clear fluids or, if
important, their usual formula.

d.  Should diarrhea follow administration of iopanoic acid, treat promptly.

e.  A chocolate fatty meal is usually given as part
of the examination.  Inform the department if
there is hypersensitivity to chocolate or other
contraindication.

f.  If necessary, the examination may be repeated
once, the next day.  Use the same dose of
iopanoic acid; do not give a "double dose."

M I S C E L L A N E O U S

1. Sweat Electrolyte Test Using Pilocarpine
   Iontophoresis

   a. Purpose:  Localized sweating induced by
      applying iontophoresis of pilocarpine to small
      skin area, and sweat collected onto filter
      paper.

   b. Method:  Each of the EKG electrodes is plugged
      to the positive or negative pole of the power
      supply.  Two squares of filter paper are cut
      (with dimensions somewhat larger than the
      electrodes) and placed over a flat skin sur-
      face (forearm, or, in infants, the thigh).  The
      papers are saturated with 0.2% pilocarpine
      nitrate and the positive electrode placed over
      the saturated papers.  It is important that
      the bare metal not touch the skin in order to
      prevent electrical burns.  The negative elec-
      trode is liberally coated with EKG paste and
      placed elsewhere on the extremity.  Each
      electrode is held gently in place by EKG
      rubber straps.

      The instrument is turned on and the current
      adjusted slowly to 2 milliamperes unless patient
      discomfort is such that the current need be
      reduced to 1 to 1.5 ma.

      After allowing the current to flow for 5
      minutes the positive electrode is removed,
      the skin rapidly washed 5 times with distilled
      water and dried thoroughly with gauze sponges.

      The weighed ash-free filter paper (obtained
      from the laboratory) is quickly removed from
      the weighing bottle with forceps and placed
      over the skin area previously covered with the
      positive electrode.  This paper is then rapidly
      covered with a plastic sheet (somewhat larger
      than the paper) and taped in place with strips
      of waterproof adhesive tape previously prepared.

      After 30 minutes the tape and plastic sheet
      are removed and the now wet paper is quickly
      placed in the weighing bottle and immediately
      returned to the laboratory where the sweat will
      be leached with appropriate diluents and
      analyzed for chloride.

    c.  Interpretation: Cystic Fibrosis associated with values of >50 mEq/L. Addison's Disease and Panhypopituitarism may also give abnormally high values.

       N.B.: The amount of chloride in the sweat test may be falsely low in children with cystic fibrosis in the face of significant edema.

       Ref: Ped. 23:545, 1959.
            New Eng. J. Med. 264:13, 1961.

2. Rapid Screening for Cold Agglutinins

    a. Method:
      1) Collect 4-5 drops of blood in a 60x7 mm Wassermann tube with approximately 0.2 ml of 3.8% sodium citrate solution.
      2) Cork tube and place in ice water.
      3) After about 30 seconds, tilt tube on its side allowing blood to run down length of tube.
      4) Definite floccular agglutination, seen with the naked eye, which disappears on warming to 37° centigrade is considered positive. Use of a control patient makes interpretation easier.

    b. Interpretation: Positives correlate with a cold agglutinin titer of 1:64 or greater.
       False positives   - almost none.
       False negatives   - about 2%

       Ref: Ann. Int. Med. 70:701, 1969.

3. Lupus Preparation

    a. Obtain 3-1/2 to 4 cc of whole blood in a heparinized Wassermann tube.
    b. Test must be run within 2 hours of drawing time. The sooner, the better.
    c. Add 5 glass beads to the blood and mix well.
    d. Rotate tube of blood, with the beads in it, for 30 minutes on the Aloe Rotator, or manually.
    e. Spin the entire sample, beads and all, at 1000-1200 rpm, for 10 minutes.
    f. Discard the plasma and lifting the buffy coat carefully, fill a Wintrobe hematocrit and spin it as the sample was spun in step (e). This should produce a large concentrated buffy coat.
    g. Discard the plasma. Gently remove the buffy coat layer and place 1 drop in a coverslip and proceed to pull smears as for peripheral blood differential.

h. Stain with Wright's for 1 minute and dilute with distilled water for 10-13 minutes.
i. Mount and examine under low dry, checking when necessary under high dry, for LE cells, rosettes, and extracellular material.
j. LE cell recognized by presence of relatively smooth, homogeneous, nuclear mass which stains a pale blue color and is less prominent than host nucleus. The latter is compressed to periphery of the cell by the cytoplasmic inclusion. The phagocytic cell is usually a polymorphonuclear leukocyte.

4. Nasal Smear for Eosinophils

   a. Method: Patient is instructed to blow nose, or collect nasal secretions by suction. Smear thinly on glass slide and dry. Stain with Giemsa, Hansel or Wright Stain. Compare number of eosinophils and neutrophils.
   b. Interpretation:
      1) Large numbers of eosinophils suggest allergy.
      2) Large numbers of neutrophils suggest infection.
      3) Eosinophils and neutrophils suggest chronic allergy with superimposed infection.

      NOTE: Large numbers of nasal eosinophils may or may not have coincidental blood eosinophilia; there is no correlation.

      Ref: Allergy in Children by Mueller, 1970, Gardner Press.

5. Peritoneal Dialysis

   a. Procedure:
      1) Patient is placed in supine position and prepped and shaved appropriately after the bladder has been emptied.
      2) Local anesthesia (1% xylocaine) is injected in the midline, down 1/3 of the distance from the umbilicus to the symphysis pubis.
      3) A small puncture is made with a #11 scalpel point in the anesthetized area down to the linea alba but not through the peritoneum.
      4) An intracath is inserted into the peritoneal cavity, and the needle removed.
      5) A quantity of warmed dialysis fluid is introduced into the peritoneal cavity sufficient to slightly distend the abdomen and allow the intestines to float.

6) The intracath is removed and the trocar with the dialysis catheter fitted over it is pushed through the existing perforation. This may require considerable force. One hand should be used to control the depth of the initial entry. The trocar is removed, and after making sure all the perforations on the dialysis catheter are within the peritoneal cavity, the catheter is cut to an appropriate length, connected to the warmed dialysis solution and the entire apparatus supported by gauze squares and covered with a dressing. The quantity of fluid for each pass is approximated on the basis of 50-75 ml/kg.

7) It should take no longer than 10 minutes to run-in each pass. The fluid should remain in the peritoneal cavity 30-45 minutes, and run out in 10-15 minutes.

8) 24-36 passes has been used as a standard number.

9) All fluid should be warmed to 37° C.

10) Careful records of vital signs, time and amounts of fluid in and out and cumulative deficits in either direction, must be kept with each pass. In addition electrolytes, SUN, cultures of the peritoneal fluid and patient's weight should be determined at least every 12 passes.

b. Available Fluids and Additives

1) Solution with 1.5% dextrose: Standard solution whose osmolality is 370 mOsm/L.

2) Solution with 4.5% dextrose (550 mOsm/L): Much higher osmolality for taking off large quantities of fluid rapidly. Must be used carefully and sparingly due to large fluid shifts and subsequent hypotension. Hypertonic passes should remain in the peritoneal cavity no longer than 30 minutes.

3) Heparin can be added, 500 units/L, to avoid fibrin clots on the catheter but this is not necessary.

4) K+ can be added, 3-4 mEq/L, when the patient's K+ is <4.5 mEq/L and renal function is adequate.

5) Most fluids commercially available are prepared with lactate as a bicarbonate
   precursor.  In situations where there is
   hepatic failure, metabolic acidosis, or
   lactic acidosis, a solution prepared with
   acetate is better.  Another option is to
   prepare a lactate free solution in the
   following manner:
   (Personal communication, Dr. Kenneth B.Roberts)

|         |                        |
|---------|------------------------|
| 905 ml  | 0.45 N NaCl            |
| 15 ml   | NaCl (2 mEq/ml)        |
| 50 ml   | NaHCO$_3$ (1 mEq/ml)   |
| 30 ml   | D$_{50}$W              |
| 1000 ml | (D$_{1.5}$; 150 mEq Na; 100 mEq Cl; 50 mEq HCO$_3$) |

Ref: NEJM 281: 945, 1969.
     Clin. Ped. 12:131, 1973.

PART II

FORMULARY

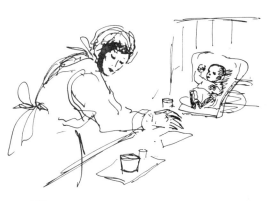

aaron Sopher

DRUG INDEX

| Trade Name | Generic Name |
|---|---|
| Aarane | Disodium Cromoglycate |
| Achromycin | Tetracycline |
| Adrenalin | Epinephrine |
| Adriamycin | Doxorubicin |
| AEP | AEP |
| Aerosporin | Polymyxin B |
| Albumin | Albumin |
| Aldactone | Spironolactone |
| Aldomet | Methyldopa |
| Alkeran | Melphalan |
| Amethopterin | Methotrexate |
| Aminophylline | Aminophylline |
| Ammonium Chloride | Ammonium Chloride |
| Amoxil | Amoxicillin |
| Amytal | Amobarbital |
| Ancobon | 5-Fluorocytosine |
| Anectine | Succinylcholine |
| Ansolysin | Pentolinium |
| Antepar | Piperazine |
| Antiminth | Pyrantel |
| Apomorphine | Apomorphine |
| Apresoline | Hydralazine |
| Aqua-Mephyton | Vitamin $K_1$ |
| Ara-C | Cytosine Arabinoside |
| Aralen | Chloroquine |
| Aramine | Metaraminol |
| L-Asparginase | L-Asparginase |
| Aspirin | Acetylsalicylic Acid |
| Atabrine | Quinacrine |
| Atarax | Hydroxyzine |
| Atropine | Atropine |
| Azulfidine | Salicylazosulfapyridine |
| Bactrim | Trimethoprim Sulfamethoxazole |
| BCNU | Carmustine |
| Belladonna Tincture | Belladonna Tincture |
| Benadryl | Diphenhydramine |
| Bleomycin | Bleomycin |
| Busulfan | Alkyl-Sulfate |
| Calcium Chloride | Calcium Chloride |
| Calcium Gluconate | Calcium Gluconate |
| Calcium Lactate | Calcium Lactate |
| Celontin | Methsuximide |
| Chloromycetin | Chloramphenicol |
| Chlor-Trimetron | Chlorpheniramine |
| Cleocin | Clindamycin |
| Codeine | Codeine |
| Colace | Dioctyl Sodium Sulfo-succinate |

| | |
|---|---|
| Coly-Mycin | Colistin |
| Compazine | Prochlorperazine |
| Corticosteroids | Corticosteroids |
| | (see table) |
| Corticotropin | ACTH |
| Cosmegen | Actinomycin D |
| Cuprimine | Penicillamine |
| Cytomel | Triiodothyronine |
| Cytosar | Cytosine Arabinoside |
| Cytoxan | Cyclophosphamide |
| Daunomycin | Daunorubicin |
| Darvon | Propoxyphene |
| Dactinomycin | Actinomycin D |
| Declomycin | Demethylchlortetracycline |
| Demerol | Meperidine |
| Dexedrine | Dextroamphetamine |
| Diamox | Acetazolamide |
| Digitalis | Digitalis |
| | (see table) |
| Dilantin | Diphenylhydantoin |
| Diuril | Chlorothiazide |
| Dulcolax | Bisacodyl |
| Dynapen | Dicloxacillin |
| Edecrin | Ethacrynic Acid |
| Elixophyllin | Theophylline |
| Ephedrine | Ephedrine |
| Epsom Salts | Magnesium Sulfate |
| Equanil | Meprobamate |
| Erythrocin | Erythromycin |
| Ferrous Gluconate | Iron Salts |
| Ferrous Sulfate | Iron Salts |
| Flagyl | Metronidazole |
| 5-FU | 5-Fluorouracil |
| Fulvicin | Griseofulvin |
| Fungizone | Amphotericin B |
| Furadantin | Nitrofurantoin |
| Gantrisin | Sulfisoxazole |
| Garamycin | Gentamicin |
| Geopen | Carbenicillin |
| Glucagon | Glucagon |
| Grifulvin | Griseofulvin |
| Grisactin | Griseofulvin |
| Halotex | Haloprogin |
| Hetrazan | Diethylcarbamazine |
| Hyoscine | Scopolamine |
| Hyperstat | Diazoxide |
| Ilosone | Erythromycin |
| Imferon | Iron Dextran |
| Imuran | Azathioprine |
| Inderal | Propranolol |
| INH | Isoniazid |
| Insulin | Insulin |
| | (see table) |

| | |
|---|---|
| Intal | Disodium Cromoglycate |
| Ipecac | Ipecac |
| Ismelin | Guanethidine |
| Isuprel | Isoproterenol |
| Kantrex | Kanamycin |
| Kaon | Potassium Gluconate |
| Kayexalate | Sodium Polystyrene Sulfonate |
| Keflex | Cephalexin |
| Keflin | Cephalothin |
| Kefzol | Cephazolin |
| Konakion | Vitamin $K_1$ |
| Kwell | Gamma Benzene Hexachloride |
| Lasix | Furosemide |
| Levophed | Levarterenol |
| Leucovorin | Leucovorin |
| Leukeran | Chlorambucil |
| Lincocin | Lincomycin |
| Liquaemin | Heparin |
| Lomidine | Pentamidine |
| Luminal | Phenobarbital |
| Lytic Cocktail | Lytic Cocktail |
| Magnesium Sulfate | Magnesium Sulfate |
| Mandelamine | Methenamine Mandelate |
| Mannitol | Mannitol |
| Matulane | Procarbazine |
| Mecholyl | Methacholine |
| Mercuhydrin | Meralluride |
| Mesantoin | Mephenytoin |
| Methylene Blue | Methylene Blue |
| Milk of Magnesia | Magnesium Hydroxide Suspension |
| Miltown | Meprobamate |
| Minocin | Minocycline |
| Mintezol | Thiabendazole |
| Mithracin | Mithramycin |
| Morphine | Morphine |
| Myambutal | Ethambutol |
| Mycostatin | Nystatin |
| Myleran | Alkyl-sulfonate |
| Mysoline | Primidone |
| Nalline | Nalorphine |
| Narcan | Naloxone |
| Nembutal | Pentobarbital |
| Neomycin | Neomycin |
| Neocalglucon | Calcium Glucogalacto-gluconate |
| Neosporin | Neomycin |
| Neo-Synephrine | Phenylephrine |
| Nitrogen Mustard | Nitrogen Mustard |
| Noctec | Chloral Hydrate |

| | |
|---|---|
| Omnipen | Ampicillin |
| Oncovin | Vincristine |
| Pamisyl | p-Aminosalicylic Acid |
| Paraldehyde | Paraldehyde |
| Paregoric | Paregoric |
| PAS | p-Aminosalicylic Acid |
| Pathocil | Dicloxacillin |
| Pavulon | Pancuronium |
| Penicillin | Penicillin |
| Periactin | Cyproheptadine |
| Phenergan | Promethazine |
| Phytonadione | Vitamin $K_1$ |
| Pilocar | Pilocarpine |
| Pitressin | Vasopressin |
| Polycillin | Ampicillin |
| Polycitra | Oral Citrate Solution |
| Potassium Chloride | Potassium Supplements |
| Potassium Gluconate | Potassium Supplements |
| Potassium Iodide | Potassium Iodide |
| Potassium Triplex | Potassium Supplements |
| Povan | Pyrivinium |
| Pro-Banthine | Propantheline |
| Pronestyl | Procainamide |
| Prostigmin | Neostigmine |
| Protamine | Protamine |
| PTU | Propylthiouracil |
| Purinethol | Mercaptopurine |
| Pyopen | Carbenicillin |
| Pyribenzamine | Tripelennamine |
| Pyridium | Phenazopyridine |
| Quinidine | Quinidine |
| Regitine | Phentolamine |
| Rimactane | Rifampin |
| Ritalin | Methylphenidate |
| Robaxin | Methocarbamol |
| Rubidomycin | Daunorubicin |
| L-Sarcolysin | Melphalan |
| Seconal | Secobarbital |
| Serpasil | Reserpine |
| Spectra | Trimethoprim-Sulfamethoxazole |
| SSKI | Potassium Iodide |
| Staphcillin | Methicillin |
| Steroids | Corticosteroids (see table) |
| Streptomycin | Streptomycin |
| Sudafed | Pseudoephedrine |
| Sulamyd | Sulfacetamide |
| Sulfadiazine | Sulfadiazine |
| Sultrin | Sulfathiazole |
| Sus-phrine | Epinephrine |
| Synthroid | Levothyroxine |
| Tapazole | Methimazole |

| | |
|---|---|
| Tedral | Tedral |
| Tegopen | Cloxacillin |
| Tempra | Acetaminophen |
| Tensilon | Edrophonium |
| THAM | Tromethamine |
| 6-Thioguanine | 6-Thioguanine |
| Thiomerin | Mercaptomerin |
| Thiotepa | Ethylenimines |
| Thorazine | Chlorpromazine |
| Thyroid | Thyroid |
| Tigan | Trimethobenzamide |
| Tinactin | Tolnaftate |
| Tofranil | Imipramine |
| TPSA | Ethylenimines |
| Trichofuron | Furazolidone |
| TRIS | Tromethamine |
| Tridione | Trimethadione |
| Tylenol | Acetaminophen |
| Unipen | Nafcillin |
| Valium | Diazepam |
| Velban | Vinblastine |
| Veracillin | Dicloxacillin |
| Vibramycin | Doxycycline |
| Vistaril | Hydroxyzine |
| Xylocaine | Lidocaine |
| Yomesan | Niclosamide |
| Zarontin | Ethosuximide |
| Zyloprim | Allopurinol |

DRUG DOSES

| Drug | Supplied | Dose and Route | Remarks |
|------|----------|----------------|---------|
| Acetaminophen (Tylenol) (Tempra) | Tablets: 120 + 325 mg<br>Syrup: 120 mg/5 ml<br>Drops: 60 mg/0.6 ml<br>Supp: 300 mg, 600 mg | <1 yr: 60 mg q4-6h PO<br><3 yr: 120 mg q4-6h PO<br>>3 yr: 120-240 mg q4-6h PO<br>Adult: 0.3-0.6 gm TID | |
| Acetazolamide (Diamox) | Tablets: 125 + 250 mg<br>Vials: 500 mg | 10-30 mg/kg/day PO divided q6-8h | Parasthesias, polyuria. For use in salicylate poisoning see page 213 |
| Acetylsalicylic Acid (Aspirin) | Tablets: 75 + 300 mg<br>Supp: 60, 300, 600 mg | Antipyretic: 30-60 mg/kg/day PO divided q4-6h<br>Antirheumatic: 100 mg/Kg/day PO divided q4-6h | Use with caution in infants. When used as antirheumatic follow serum levels and observe for intoxication. Probably contraindicated in platelid disorders. |
| ACTH (Corticotropin) | Aqueous: 40 units/5 ml<br>Gel: 40 + 80 units/5 ml | Aqueous: 1.6 units/kg/day IV, IM or SC divided q6-8h<br>Gel: 0.8 units/kg/day divided q12h IM. | Contraindicated in acute psychoses, Cushing's Syndrome, active TBC or peptic ulcer. |

| | | | |
|---|---|---|---|
| Actinomycin D (Cosmegen) (Dactinomycin) | Vials: 0.5 mg | I.V. | Cellulitis with extravasation, nausea, vomiting, alopecia, stomatitis, "flare reaction" to previously irradiated areas (including internal organs). *Bone marrow depression |
| Adriamycin | Vials: 10 mg | I.V. | Nausea, vomiting, stomatitis, alopecia, "red urine" phlebitis, cellulitis with extravasation *Bone marrow depression *Cardiac toxicity with cumulative dose >550 mg/m2 |
| AEP Tablets | Tablets: aminophylline 100 mg ephedrine 16 mg phenobarbital 16 mg (all per tablet) | 1 tab/10 kg/day divided q6-8h PO | Dose limited by aminophylline content of tablet. |
| Albumin | Vials: 5 gm/20 ml 25 gm/100 ml | 0.5-1.0 gm/kg/dose IV | Use with caution in hypervolemic states. |

*Dose limiting side effects

| | | | |
|---|---|---|---|
| Allopurinol (Zyloprim) | Tablets: 100 mg | 10 mg/kg/day divided q8h PO | Use in children limited to hyperuricemia of malignancies. Establish alkaline urine flow. |
| Alkyl-Sulfonate (Myleran) (Busulfan) | Tablets: 2 mg | PO | Skin pigmentation, gynecomastia, chelosis, glossitis, anhidrosis, pulmonary fibrosis. *Bone marrow depression. |
| Aminophylline | Ampules: 25 mg/ml (10 ml ampule) Tablets: 100 + 200 mg Supp: 125, 250, + 500 mg | 2-5 mg/kg/dose PO q8h PRN Status Asthmaticus: 5-6 mg/kg over 15-20 min. IV, then 0.9 mg/kg/hr continuous IV infusion Ref: NEJM 289: 600, 1973 | Potentiates effect of epinephrine. IV infusion over 5-15 minutes. Suppositories not recommended for treatment of status asthmaticus. |
| Ammonium Chloride | Tablets: 500 mg Vials: 4 mEq/ml | 75 mg/kg/day PO divided q6h 2-6 gm/day PO for diuresis or acidification of urine | Continued use may cause acidosis. Use with caution in infants or in liver disease. |
| Amobarbital (Amytal) | Tablets: 30, 50, 100 mg Capsules: 200 mg Ampules: 250 + 500 mg | Sedation: 6 mg/kg/day PO divided q8h | Use with caution in hepatic disease, CNS or respiratory depression. |

*Dose limiting side effects

| Drug | Form | Dosage | Comments |
|---|---|---|---|
| Amoxicillin (Amoxil) | Capsules: 250 mg + 500 mg. Suspension: 125 mg + 250 mg/5 ml. Pediatric drops: 50 mg/ml | 20-50 mg/kg/day PO divided q8h (Max. daily dose 12 gm) | Less G.I. side effects, otherwise same as Ampicillin except not indicated for Shigella. |
| Amphotericin B (Fungizone) | Vials: 50 mg | Test Dose: 0.1 mg/kg on first day of therapy IV over 6 hours. Then Increase to: 1 mg/kg/day IV as single infusion over 6-8 hours. | Do not use if precipitate present in solution. Local and systemic reactions common. Follow hepatic, renal and hematopoietic indices closely. |
| Ampicillin (Polycillin) (Omnipen) | Capsules: 250 + 500 mg. Susp: 125 + 250 mg/5 ml. Vials: 250, 500 mg, 1 gm | 50-400 mg/kg/day PO, IM or IV divided q6h. <1 week 50-100 mg/kg/day q12h. 1-4 wks. 100-200 mg/kg/day q8h. (Max. dose = 12 gm/day) | Same side reactions as penicillin, with allergic cross-reactivity. 2.7 mEq Na/gm ampicillin |
| Apomorphine | Vials: 10 mg/ml | Emetic Dose: 0.1 mg/kg/dose IM or SC | Decomposed solution turns green. Use cautiously in sedated patients. |

132

| | | | |
|---|---|---|---|
| L-Asparaginase | Vials: 10,000 IU + 50,000 IU (refrigerate) | IV | Fever, nausea, vomiting, hepatotoxic, prolonged prothrombin & partial thromboplastin time, decreased fibrinogen, somonolence, tremors. *Hypersensitivity reaction with anaphylaxis. *Pancreatitis, *Hyperglycemia, *Seizures. |
| Atropine | Tablets: 0.32, 0.4, 0.65 mg<br>Vials: 1 mg/ml<br>Ophthalmic Solution: 0.5, 1, 3%<br>Ophthalmic Ointment: 1% | 0.01 mg/kg/dose PO or SC q4-6h PRN (Max. single dose = 0.4 mg) | Children with Down's Syndrome may be hypersensitive. Contraindicated in glaucoma. See PREANESTHETIC MEDICATION on page 196 |
| Azathioprine (Imuran) | Tablets: 50 mg | Initial: 3-5 mg/kg/day PO Maintenance: may be reduced to 1-2 mg/kg/day PO according to patient's response. | Blood dyscrasias not infrequent. Follow hematologic, GI, and hepatic function closely, especially in presence of renal disease. |

*Dose limiting side effects

| Drug | Preparation | Dose | Side effects |
|---|---|---|---|
| BCNU (Carmustine) | Vials: 100 mg (refrigerate) Oral—CCNU Capsules: 50 + 100 mg | PO | Nausea, vomiting, jaundice, flushing of face, phlebitis with pain on IV administration. *Leucopenia & thrombocytopenia delayed 4-6 weeks. |
| Belladonna Tincture | Dropper Bottles: 30 + 60 ml (1 ml approximately = 0.3 mg atropine) | 0.1 ml/kg/day PO divided q6-8h (Max. total dose = 3.5 ml/day) | Toxicity same as atropine. |
| Bleomycin | Vials: 15 units | IV | Skin toxicity, nausea, vomiting, fever. *Pulmonary fibrosis with >400 units. |
| Bisacodyl (Dulcolax) | Tablets: 5 mg (enteric) Supp: 10 mg | 0.3 mg/kg/dose PO 6 hours before desired effect. | Do not chew tablets. Not recommended for newborn. |
| Calcium Chloride (27% calcium) | Ampules: 10% (100 mg/ml) (14 mEq Ca/gm salt: 73 mg salt/mEq Ca | 250-300 mg/kg/day PO as 2% solution divided q6h | Irritating IV and on GI tract. Acidifying: give 2-3 days then change to another salt. |

*Dose limiting side effects

| Drug | Preparation | Dose | Comments |
|---|---|---|---|
| Calcium Gulconate (9% calcium) Calcium Gluco-galactogluco-nate (Neocalglucon) | Tablets (gluconate): 1 gm Ampules (gluconate): 10% (100 mg/ml) (4 mEq Ca/gm salt: 224 mg salt/mEq Ca) Syrup (Neocalglucon): 4 ml = 1 gm Ca glu-conate (90 mg Ca/gm salt) | 500 mg/kg/day PO in divided doses. 200 mg/kg/dose IV slowly. | If given IV, watch for bradycardia and extra-vasation. MONITOR PULSE. |
| Calcium Lactate (13% calcium) | Tablets: 600 mg (6 mEq Ca/gm salt: 154 mg salt/mEq Ca) | 500 mg/kg/day PO in divided doses. | Tablets do not dissolve in milk. |
| Carbenicillin (Geopen) (Pyopen) | Vials: 1 + 5 gm | 400-600 mg/kg/day IM or IV divided q4h (Max. adult dose: 30 gm/day) | Interaction with gen-tamycin unpredictable. Give through separate IV tubing. Rapid re-sistance when used alone. |
| Cephalexin (Keflex) | Capsules: 250 mg Oral Susp: 125 mg/5 ml | 25-50 mg/kg/day PO divided q6h (Max. dose = 4 gm/day) | GI disturbances fre-quent. Cross sensiti-vity with penicillins. Not recommended for newborn. |

| | | | |
|---|---|---|---|
| Cephalothin (Keflin) | Vials: 1 gm/10 cc<br>2 gm/100 cc<br>4 gm/50 cc | 40-150 mg/kg/day q4-6h | See Keflex. |
| Cephazolin (Kefzol) | Vials: 250 mg/5 cc<br>500 mg/5 cc<br>1 gm/10 cc | 25-100 mg/kg/day q6-8h | See Keflex. |
| Chloral Hydrate (Noctec) | Capsules: 250 + 500 mg<br>Syrup: 500 mg/5 ml<br>Supp: 300, 600 mg, 1 gm | 10-20 mg/kg/dose PO or PR repeat q6-8h PRN.<br>(Max. total dose = 50 mg/kg/day PO or PR)<br>(Max. single dose: 2.0 gm PO or PR) | Irritating to tracheo-bronchial membranes; may cause laryngospasm if aspirated. |
| Chlorambucil (Leukeran) | Tablets: 2 mg | PO | Nausea, vomiting, diarrhea, hepatotoxicity; *Bone marrow depression |
| Chloramphenicol (Chloromycetin) | Capsules: 100 + 250 mg<br>Susp: 150 mg/5 ml<br>Vials: 1 gm<br>Otic solution: 0.5%<br>Ophthalmic solution: 0.16, 0.25, 0.5%<br>Ophthalmic ointment: 1% | Prematures and Newborns: 25 mg/kg/day PO, IM or IV<br>Infants >2 wks: 50-100 mg/kg/day PO, IM or IV<br>All divided q6h<br>(Max. dose: 2 gm/day) | Adjust newborn dose according to blood levels (10-20 micrograms/ml). Follow hematologic status carefully. |

*Dose limiting side effects.

| Drug | Forms | Dosage | Comments |
|---|---|---|---|
| Chloroquine Phosphate (Aralen) | Tablets: 250 mg | Amebic Hepatitis: 10 mg/kg/day q12h PO x 14 days | Numerous toxic side effects. Severe infections and hepatic abscess may require higher doses. |
| Chlorothiazide (Diuril) | Tablets: 250 + 500 mg Susp: 250 mg/5 ml Vials: 500 mg | Infants <6 mos. 20-30 mg/kg/day PO q12h Children >6 mos: 20 mg/kg/day PO divided q12h | Use with caution in liver and severe renal disease. Follow electrolytes. May cause hyperbilirubinemia and hyperglycemia. |
| Chlorpheniramine (Chlor-Trimeton) | Tablets: 4 mg Repetabs: 8 + 12 mg Syrup: 2.5 mg/5 ml Injection: 100 mg/ml | 0.35 mg/kg/day PO or SC divided q6h | Usual side effects of antihistamines; use with caution in presence of other depressants. |
| Chlorpromazine (Thorazine) | Tablets: 10, 25, 50, 100 mg Spansules: 30, 75, 150, 200, 300 mg Syrup: 10 mg/5 ml Supp: 25 + 100 mg Oral Concentrate: 30 mg/ml Ampules: 25 mg/ml | 2 mg/kg/day PO or IM divided q6h PRN | Extrapyramidal symptoms, especially dyskinetic reactions, common. May potentiate effects of narcotics, sedatives, and other drugs. SEE LYTIC COCTAIL on page 153 |

137

| | | | |
|---|---|---|---|
| Clindamycin (Cleocin) | Capsules: 75 + 150 mg Oral Liquid: 75 mg/5 ml Vials: 150 mg/ml | 10-20 mg/kg/day PO divided q6-8h 10-40 mg/kg/day IM, IV q6h. (Max. dose = 5 gm/day) | Not indicated for infants and newborns. May cause colitis. |
| Cloxacillin (Tegopen) | Capsule: 250 mg Oral solution: 125 mg/ 5 ml | 50-200 mg/kg/day PO divided q6h (Max. dose = 6-8 gm/day) | Same side reactions as penicillins. Better absorbed PO than oxacillin. |
| Codeine | Tablets: 15, 30, 60 mg Ampules: 30 + 60 mg Elixir terpin hydrate and codeine: 10 mg codeine/5 ml | Pain: 0.5-1.0 mg/kg/dose PO or SC, repeat q4-6h PRN (usual total daily dose = 3 mg/kg/day) Cough: 0.2 mg/kg/dose PO repeat q4h PRN | May be habit forming. |
| Colistin (Coly-Mycin) | Oral Susp: 25 mg/5 ml Vials: 150 mg | Enterocolitis: 5-15 mg/ kg/day PO divided q8h Systemic: 1.5-5.0 mg/kg/ day deep IM divided q6-12h. | Use with caution in presence of renal disease. May be neurotoxic. |
| Corticosteroids | See following table on page 192-194 | | |

| Cyclophospha-mide (Cytoxan) | Tablets: 25 + 50 mg<br>Vials: 100, 200, 500 mg | PO, IV | Cellulitis on extra-vasation, vomiting alopecia.<br>*Hemorrhagic cystitis,<br>*Bone marrow depression especially leukopenia. |
| Cyproheptadine (Periactin) | Tablets: 5 mg<br>Syrup: 2 mg/5 ml | 0.25 mg/kg/day PO divided q6-8h | |
| Cytosine Arabinoside (Cytosar) (Ara-C) | Vials: 100 + 500 mg | IV | Vomiting, fever, skin rash, hepatotoxic,<br>*Bone marrow depression. |
| Daunorubicin (Daunomycin) (Rubidomycin) | Vials: 20 mg | IV | Cellulitis on extra-vasation, nausea, vomiting, fever,alope-cia,"red urine", skin rash,<br>*Bone marrow depression<br>*Cardiac toxicity with cumulative dosage $\geq 500$ mg/m$^2$. |

*Dose limiting side effects

| | | | |
|---|---|---|---|
| Demethylchlor-tetracycline (Declomycin) | Tablets: 300 mg<br>Capsules: 150 mg<br>Syrup: 75 mg/5 ml | 10 mg/kg/day PO divided q6-12h (Max. adult dose=1.2 gm/day) | See Tetracycline. |
| Dextroamphe-tamine (Dexedrine) | Tablets: 5 mg<br>Elixir: 5 mg/5 ml<br>Spansule: 10 + 15 mg | 2-15 mg/day PO divided into 2 or 3 doses or as single sustained-action dose | Use with caution in presence of hypertension or cardiovascular disease. |
| Diazepam (Valium) | Tablets: 2, 5, 10 mg<br>Ampules: 5 mg/1 ml | Sedative and muscle relaxant: 0.1-0.8 mg/kg/day PO divided q6-8h; 0.04-0.20 mg/kg/dose IM or IV slowly; repeat q2-4h PRN<br>Acute Anticonvulsant: 0.5-0.75 mg/kg. Slow IV infusion may repeat x 2 q15 min. (Max. dose = 5 mg in infants and small children and 15 mg in older children) | Use with caution in glaucoma, shock, and severely depressed patients. Acute dis-continuance may cause withdrawal symptoms 48-72 hrs. later. May cause hypotension and respiratory depression. Not good maintenance drug alone for seizures. |
| Diazoxide (Hyperstat) | Ampules: 300 mg | Hypertensive Crisis: 2-10 mg/kg/dose, rapid IV push, PRN (usually 5 mg/kg IV q2-5h) | May cause hyperglycemia, ketoacidosis, GI dis-turbances, arrhythmias, hyponatremia, hyperuri-cemia. Not yet released for children. |

140

| | | |
|---|---|---|
| Dicloxacillin (Dynapen) (Veracillin) (Pathocil) | Capsules: 125 + 250 mg Oral Susp: 62.5 mg/5 ml | 25-100 mg/kg/day PO divided q6h (dosage in newborn not established) (Max. adult dose=4 gm/day) | Allergic cross-sensitivity with penicillin. Similar toxicity and side effects to cloxacillin. |
| Diethylcarbamazine (Hetrazan) | Tablets: 50 mg Syrup: 120 mg/5 ml | Ascariasis: 15 mg/kg/day PO as single daily dose for 4 consecutive days. | |
| Digitalis | See following table on pages 184-185 | | |
| Dioctyl Sodium Sulfosuccinate (Colace) | Capsules: 50 + 100 mg Solution: 10 mg/ml Syrup: 20 mg/5 ml | 5 mg/kg/day PO divided q6-8h. | |
| Diphenhydramine (Benadryl) | Capsules: 25 + 50 mg Elixir: 12.5 mg/5 ml Ampules: 50 mg/ml Vials: 10 mg/ml | 5 mg/kg/day PO or IM divided q6h (Max. total dose = 300 mg/day) 2 mg/kg IV slowly for anaphylaxis and phenothiazine overdose. | Side effects common to antihistamines. |

| Diphenylhydantoin (Dilantin) | Capsules: 30 + 100 mg  Tablets: 50 mg  Susp: 125 mg/5 ml  Vials: 20 + 50 mg/ml | Maintenance Anticonvulsant: 5-7 mg/kg/day PO or IV (use with caution IV) divided into one or two daily doses. See Anti-arrhythmia and Anti-convulsant sections, pages 186 and 189. | Side reactions include gingival hyperplasia, dermatitis, blood dyscrasias, ataxia, lymphadenopathy and liver damage. |
| Disodium Cromoglycate (Intal) (Aarane) | Capsule: 20 mg | Inhalant 20 mg q6h | Not for acute asthma attack, must take for 2-4 weeks for adequate therapeutic trial. |
| Doxorubicin HCl (Adriamycin) | Vials: 10 mg | IV | Nausea, vomiting, stomatitis, alopecia, "red urine", phlebitis and cellulitis with extravasation. *Bone marrow depression *Cardiac toxicity with cumulative dosage >550 mg/m2 and occasionally at lower dosages. |

*Dose limiting side effects

| | | | |
|---|---|---|---|
| Doxycycline (Vibramycin) | Capsules: 50 + 100 mg Oral solution: 125 mg/ 5 ml | Initial: <45 kg: 5 mg/kg/ day PO divided q12 x 1 da. >45 kg: 200 mg/day PO divided q12h x 1 day Maintenance: <45 kg: 2.5 mg/kg/day PO single daily dose. >45 kg: 100 mg/day PO single daily dose. (Max. adult dose=200 mg/ day) | Hepatic toxicity reported. Use with caution in renal disease. See Tetracycline. |
| Edrophonium (Tensilon) | Ampules: 10 mg/ml | 0.2 mg/kg/dose IV (Max. total dose 5-10 mg). Give 1/5 of test dose IV slowly, if no response in 1 minute, give additional 1 mg increments. | Keep atropine available in syringe. May precipitate cholinergic crisis, arrhythmias, and bronchospasm. Not recommended for infants. |
| Ephedrine | Tablets: 25 + 50 mg Syrup: 4 mg/ml Capsules: 25 + 50 mg Ampules: 50 mg/ml | 0.5-1.0 mg/kg/dose PO or SC. 0.2 mg/kg/dose IM. Repeat q4-6h PRN (Max. daily dose = 3 mg/kg) | May precipate arryhth- mias and potentiate theophylline. IV drip = 50 mg/1000 ml, adjust rate to patient's response. |

| | | | |
|---|---|---|---|
| Epinephrine (Adrenalin) | 1:1000 (Aqueous) Ampules: 1 ml (1 mg/ml) Vials: 30 ml (1 mg/ml) 1:500 (in oil) Ampules: 1 ml (2 mg/ml) 1:200 (Susphrine) Vials: 5 ml (5 mg/ml) | 1:1000 (Aqueous): 0.01 ml/kg/dose SC (Max. single dose = 0.5 ml), repeat q15-20 minutes x 3-4 or q4h PRN 1:500 (In Oil): 0.01-0.02 ml/kg/dose IM, repeat q12-24h PRN 1:200 Susphrine: 0.005 ml/kg/dose SC, repeat q8-12h PRN (Max. single dose = 0.15 ml) | May produce arrhythmias, hypertension, headaches, nausea, vomiting. |
| Erythromycin Salts (Erythrocin) (Ilosone) | Erythromycin: Tablets: 125 + 250 mg Erythromycin Ethyl Succinate: Suspension: 200 mg/5 ml Erythromycin Lactobionate: Vials: 500 mg + 1 gm Erythromycin Estolate (Ilosone): Capsules: 125 + 250 mg Susp: 125 mg/5 ml | Erythromycin + Salts: Oral: 30-50 mg/kg/day divided q4-6h Parenteral: 10 mg/kg/day IM or IV divided q8-12h Erythromycin Estolate: Oral: <11 kg 40-80 mg/kg/day; 11-23 kg 0.5-1 gm/day; >23 kg 1-2 gm/day all divided q6h (Max. adult dose = 2 gm/day) | GI side effects common. use with caution in liver disease. Rheumatic Fever Prophylaxis: 200 mg/day PO. |

| Drug | Preparations | Dose | Cautions |
|---|---|---|---|
| Ethacrynic Acid (Edecrin) | Tablets: 25 + 50 mg<br>Vials: 50 mg | Children: 25 mg/dose PO, 0.5-1 mg/kg/dose IV | Ototoxicity may occur in renal disease. Caution in liver disease and severe cardiac disease. |
| Ethambutol (Myambutol) | Tablets: 100 + 400 mg | 15-25 mg/kg PO, as single daily dose. | Macular degeneration. Follow visual activity. |
| Ethosuximide (Zarontin) | Capsules: 250 mg<br>Syrup: 250 mg/5 ml | Initial Dose:<br><6 yrs: 250 mg/day PO as single dose<br>>6 yrs: 500 mg/day PO divided q12h<br>Subsequent Dose: Increase by 250 mg increments q4-7 days | Caution in liver and renal disease. May cause blood dyscrasias, GI, neurologic, and dermatologic reactions. Increase as necessary to control symptoms short of significant side effects. |
| Ethylenimines (TPSA) (Thiotepa) | Tablets: 1 + 5 mg<br>Vials: 15 mg | PO and IV | *Bone marrow depression. |
| 5-Fluorocytosine (Ancobon) | Capsules: 250 + 500 mg | 50-150 mg/kg/day q6h | Use with caution in renal failure, may cause bone marrow depression, nausea, and vomiting. |

*Dose limiting side effects

| | | | |
|---|---|---|---|
| 5-Fluorouracil (5-FU) | Vial: 500 mg | IV | Stomatitis, nausea vomiting, diarrhea, GI ulcerations, cerebellar signs. *Bone marrow depression. |
| Furazolidone & Nifuroximine (Trichofuron) | Vaginal Supp: 2 gm | 1-2 supp. qhs x 12 days | Mixed fungal and bacterial vaginal infections. |
| Furosemide (Lasix) | Tablets: 20 + 40 mg Ampules: 10 mg/ml | 0.5-1 mg/kg/dose PO, IM or IV | Ototoxicity may occur in renal disease. Give with caution in hepatic disease. |
| Gamma Benzene Hexachloride (Kwell) | Shampoo: 1% (60cc bottle) Lotion: 1% | Shampoo with 30cc; repeat in 24 hours | For pediculosis. |

*Dose limiting side effects

| Drug | Preparation | Dosage | Notes |
|---|---|---|---|
| Gentamicin (Garamycin) | Vials: 10 + 40 mg/ml | <ins>≤1 week:</ins> 5 mg/kg/day q12h IM or IV <br> <ins>1-6 weeks:</ins> 7.5 mg/kg/day q8h IM or IV <br> <ins>>6 weeks:</ins> 5.0-7.5 mg/kg day q6h IM or IV <br> Intrathecal: 1-2 mg IT q day until CSF sterile (IV dosage given slowly over 30 min.) <br><br> Ref: <ins>J. Inf. Dis.</ins> <ins>124</ins>: supp. 12/71 | Use only for life-threatening infections in infants and newborns. Monitor closely for renal and ototoxicity. Follow with serum levels. |
| Glucagon | Ampules: 1 mg/ml | <ins>General Causes of Hypoglycemia:</ins> 0.025-0.1 mg/kg/dose SC, IM, or IV. May repeat q20 min PRN (Max. total dose = 1 mg) <br> <ins>Symptomatic Infants of Diabetic Mothers:</ins> 0.30 mg/kg/dose SC, IM or IV | Do not rely on glucagon alone to correct prolonged or profound hypoglycemia in newborns; use glucose IV in addition. |
| Griseofulvin (Grifulvin) Griseofulvin Microcrystalline (Grifulvin V) (Grisactin) | Griseofulvin: Susp: 125 mg/5 ml <br> Griseofulvin Microcrystalline: Tablets: 250 + 500 mg Susp: 125 mg/5 ml | Griseofulvin: 20 mg/kg/day PO divided q6-12h <br> Griseofulvin Microcrystalline: 10 mg/kg/day PO divided q6-12h | Contraindicated in porphyria and severe hepatic disease. Absorption improved if taken with milk. Follow CBC. |

| Drug | Dosage Form | Dose | Comments |
|---|---|---|---|
| Guanethidine (Ismelin) | Tablets: 10 + 25 mg | 0.2 mg/kg/day PO as single daily dose; increase as necessary q7-10 days by 0.2 mg/kg/day increments | Contraindicated in pheochromocytoma or presence of MAO inhibitors. Caution in renal, CNS or cardiovascular disease. Postural hypotension. |
| Haloprogin (Halotex) | Cream: 1% Solution: 1% | Topically BID x 2-3 wks. | Keep away from eyes. Discontinue with increased local irritation |
| Heparin (Liquaemin) | Vials: 1000 + 10,000 units/ml Repository injection: 20,000 units/ml (120 units = approximately 1 mg) | Initial Dose: 50 units/kg IV drip Maintenance Dose: 100 units/kg/dose IV drip, repeat q4h | Titrate dose to give clotting time of 20-30 minutes or 2-3 times normal, immediately before each dose. Antidote: Protamine Sulfate. |
| Hydralazine (Apresoline) | Tablets: 10, 25, 50 + 100 mg Ampules: 20 mg/ml | Oral: 0.75 mg/kg/day divided q6h (may increase slowly over 3-4 wks. to max. dose of 7.5 mg/kg/day) Parenteral Alone: 1.7-3.5 mg/kg/day IM or IV divided q4-6h Parenteral with Reserpine: 0.15 mg/kg/dose IM or IV q12-24h. | Use with caution in severe renal disease. May cause lupus and and arthritic-like syndromes. |

148

| Drug | Forms | Dosage | Cautions |
|---|---|---|---|
| Hydroxyzine Salts (Atarax) (Vistaril) | Tablets: 10 mg (hydrochloride) Capsules: 25 + 50 mg (pamoate) Syrup: 25 mg/5 ml (pamoate) Vials: 50 mg/ml (hydrochloride) | 2 mg/kg/day PO divided q6-8h | May potentiate barbiturates, meperidine, and other depressants. |
| Imipramine (Tofranil) | Tablets: 10, 25, 50 mg Vials: 12.5 mg/ml | Sedative: 1.5 mg/kg/day PO or IM divided q6-8h Enuresis: 10-75 mg PO qhs Max dose: 5-6 yrs.-40 mg 6-8 yrs. -50 mg 8-10 yrs.-60 mg 10-12 yrs.-70 mg 12-14 yrs.-75 mg<br><br>Ref: PCNA 21:1024, 1974 | Caution in presence of glaucoma, cardiac arrhythmias, MAO inhibitors. |
| Insulin | See table on page 190 | | |
| Ipecac | Syrup: 0.14% alkaloids | >1 yr: 15 ml PO followed with water; may repeat in 15-20 minutes once if needed. | NEVER use FLUID EXTRACT of Ipecac. May be fatal. |

149

| | Preparation | Total Dose in mg Fe | Comments |
|---|---|---|---|
| Iron Dextran (Imferon) | Ampules: 2 ml<br>Vials: 10 ml<br>(50 mg elemental Fe/ml) | Total Dose in mg Fe:<br>Surface area (M2) x 55 x (13.5 - Hgb in gm%) = mg Fe needed IM. May add 10-50% for stores. Give 1-2 ml/day until total dose given. | Use "Z" technique of IM administration. Numerous side effects and toxic reactions including anaphylaxis. Inject test dose of 0.1-0.2 ml the first day. |
| Iron Salts | Ferrous Sulfate:<br>Oral liquid (drops) - (Fer-in-Sol): 125 mg FeSO4/ml = 25 mg Fe/ml<br>Syrup (elixir) - (Feosol): 40 mg FeSO4/ml = 8 mg Fe/ml<br>Tablets: 300 mg FeSO4 = 60 mg Fe<br>Ferrous Gluconate: (Fergon)<br>Oral liquid (elixir): 60 mg Fe gluconate/ml = 7 mg Fe/ml<br>Tablets: 300 mg Fe gluconate = 35 mg Fe | Treatment: 6 mg Fe/kg/day PO divided q8h.<br>Prophylaxis:<br>Prematures, newborns, and infants predisposed to anemia: 8-15 mg Fe/day PO divided q8-12h for first 6-12 months of life.<br>Older Infants and Children: 1 mg Fe/kg/day PO single or divided doses. | Ferrous salts better absorbed than ferric salts. Do not use in hemolytic diseases. Less absorbed when given with meals. |

| | | | |
|---|---|---|---|
| Isoniazid (INH) | Tablets: 100 mg<br>Syrup: 50 mg/5 ml<br>Ampules: 100 mg/ml | Therapeutic:<br>15-20 mg/kg/day PO or<br>10 mg/kg/day IM divided<br>q8-12h (total max. dose<br>= 300-500 mg/day)<br>Prophylactic:<br>10 mg/kg/day PO divided<br>q8-12h or single daily<br>dose if tolerated (total<br>max. dose = 300 mg/day) | CNS and hepatic side<br>effects not infrequent<br>with high dosages.<br>Slow acetylators more<br>likely to develop toxi-<br>city. Supplement<br>adolescents with pyri-<br>doxine. |
| Isoproterenol (Isuprel) | Tablets: 10 + 15 mg<br>Elixir: 2.5 mg/15 ml<br>Nebulizer: 1:100, 1:200<br>Ampules: 0.2 mg/1 ml,<br>1 mg/5 ml | Sublingual: 5-10 mg/dose<br>PO repeat q6-8h PRN<br>IV Infusion: 0.05-4.0<br>micrograms/minute; adjust<br>rate to patient's<br>response (1 ampule =<br>1 mg; therefore 1 ampule<br>in 250 ml D5W = 4 micro-<br>gram/ml)<br><br>Ref: PCNA 21:974, 976,<br>1974 | Use with care in pre-<br>sence of congestive<br>failure. May cause<br>arrhythmias in combina-<br>tion with epinephrine.<br>Monitor C.V.P., heart<br>rate, and blood pressure. |

| Drug | Form | Dose | Notes |
|---|---|---|---|
| Kanamycin (Kantrex) | Capsule: 500 mg<br>Vials: 75 mg/2 ml<br>500 mg/2 ml<br>1000 mg/3 ml | Enteric: 50 mg/kg/day PO divided q6h<br>Systemic:<br>Premature and Infants<br><1 yr: 15 mg/kg/day IM divided q12h<br>Older children: 6-15 mg/kg/day IM divided q12h.<br>(Max. adult dose = 1.5 gm/day) | Renal and auditory toxicity frequent. Avoid IV use. |
| Leucovorin | Solution: 3 mg/ml | PO, IM, IV equal to amount of methotrexate (mg for mg) within 1 hour, then 1/2 dose q6h x 12h | |
| Levarterenol Bitartrate (Levophed) | Ampules: 2 mg of bitartrate/ml (0.2%) | IV Infusion: 1 ampule = 4 ml (8 mg of bitartrate/1 liter D5W gives 8 microgram/ml) Test dose 0.2 micrograms/kg; follow by titrating dose with patient's BP. Usual rate of administration: 0.5-1.0 ml (4-8 micrograms)/minute | Treatment for extravasation: phentolamine, 5-10 mg in 15 ml saline, infiltrated locally. |

| | | |
|---|---|---|
| Levothyroxine (Synthroid) | Tablets: 50, 100, 200, 300 micrograms<br>Vials: 500 micrograms | Calculate dosage as for desiccated thyroid according to following equivalencies: 1 grain (65 mg) USP desiccated thyroid = 100 micrograms Thyroxine | See Thyroid. |
| Lidocaine (Xylocaine) | Vials: 0.5, 1, 2, 4, 5% (50 ml)<br>(1% solution = 10 mg/ml)<br>Ointment: 2.5 + 5% (35 gm tubes)<br>Susp. (viscous): 2% (100 ml)<br>Jelly: 2% (30 ml tubes) | Anesthetic: apply or infiltrate locally PRN (max. total dose 3-5 mg/kg)<br>Anti-arrhythmia: single bolus (2% solution): 0.5-1.0 mg/kg/dose slowly may repeat q5-10 min PRN. Continuous IV infusion: 20-50 micrograms/kg/min (Max. total dose=5 mg/kg) | Topical administration may facilitate allergic sensitization. Side effects of IV administration may include hypotension, seizures, cardiac asystole, and respiratory arrest. |
| Lincomycin (Lincocin) | Capsules: 250 + 500 mg<br>Syrup: 250 mg/5 ml<br>Vials: 300 mg/ml | Oral: 30-60 mg/kg/day divided q6-8h<br>Intramuscular: 10-20 mg/kg/day single dose or divided q12h<br>Intravenous: 10-20 mg/kg/day divided q8-12h (Max. adult dose = 5 gm/day) | Contraindicated in infants under 1 month of age. Use with caution in presence of liver or renal disease. |

| Drug | Preparation | Dosage | Comments |
|---|---|---|---|
| Lytic Cocktail (DPT) | | Demerol: 2 mg/kg<br>Phenergan: 1 mg/kg<br>Thorazine: 1 mg/kg<br>(Max. dose = 50 mg Demerol) | Mix in one syringe and give deep IM. |
| Magnesium Hydroxide Suspension (Milk of Magnesia) | USP magma (milk): 8% magnesium hydroxide | 0.5 ml/kg/dose PO | |
| Magnesium Sulfate | Ampules: 500 mg/ml (2 ml)<br>Oral Solution: 50% (Epsom salts) | Cathartic: 250 mg/kg/dose PO<br>Hypertension:<br>IM: 50% solution (500 mg/ml) 0.2 ml/kg/dose repeat q4-6h PRN<br>IV: 1% solution (10 mg/ml) (Max.: 100 mg/kg/dose slowly) | Monitor blood pressure and respirations. Calcium gluconate (IV) should be available as antidote. |
| Mannitol | Vials: 250 mg/ml (25%) | Test Dose: 200 mg/kg IV single dose over 3-5 min.<br>Edema: (15-20% solution) Ascites or generalized: 1-2 gm/kg IV as slow infusion over 2-6h.<br>Cerebral or Ocular: 1-2 gm/kg IV over 30-60 min. | May cause circulatory overload and electrolyte disturbances. |

154

| Drug | | | |
|---|---|---|---|
| Melphalan (Alkeran) (L-Sarcolysin) | Tablets: 2 mg | PO | *Bone marrow depression. |
| Merperidine (Demerol) | Tablets: 50 mg<br>Elixir: 50 mg/ml<br>Vials: 50 + 100 mg/ml | 6 mg/kg/day PO, IM, or SC divided q4-6h PRN (Max. single dose = 50-100 mg/dose) | Contraindicated in cardiac arrhythmias, increased intracranial pressure, and asthma. Potentiated by MAO inhibitors, phenothiazines, isoniazid, other CNS acting agents. 75 mg Demerol = 10 mg Morphine. |
| Mephenytoin (Mesantoin) | Tablets: 100 mg | 3-15 mg/kg/day PO divided q8h. Start at low dose, increase q7 days. (Max. = 200-400 mg q8h) | May cause blood dyscrasias, rash, drowsiness, ataxia. |
| Meprobamate (Equanil) (Miltown) | Tablets: 400 mg<br>Susp: 200 mg/5 ml | 25 mg/kg/day PO divided q8-12h (Adult max. = 400-800 mg/dose) | Do not discontinue abruptly because of danger of withdrawal symptoms. |

*Dose limiting side effects

155

| Meralluride (Mercuhydrin) | Ampules: 130 mg/ml (1 ml contains 39 mEq Hg + 48 mg theophylline) | 4-6 mg/kg/day or approximately:<br><15 kg: 0.04 ml/kg/day<br>15-35 kg: 0.03 mg/kg/day<br>>35 kg: 1-2 ml/day IM, as single dose, usually q2-3 days. May be given no more often than once daily (Max. dose = 2 ml) | May require K+ supplementation. Contraindicated in oliguria and nephritis. |
| Mercaptomerin (Thiomerin) | Vials: 125 mg/ml (1 ml contains 40 mg Hg) | As for meralluride | As for meralluride. |
| Mercaptopurine (Purinethol) | Tablets: 50 mg | PO | Vomiting,<br>*Bone marrow depression |
| Metaraminol (Aramine) | Vials: 10 mg/ml (10 ml) | IM: 0.1 mg/kg/dose IM or SC as single dose PRN<br>IV Single Dose: 0.01 mg/kg/dose IV PRN<br>Continuous Infusion:<br>1 ml/250 ml D5W or NS; adjust rate to maintain blood pressure. (Max. total dose = 0.4 mg/kg) | Use with caution during cyclopropane anesthesia, in thyroid or heart disease, or in diabetes. |

*Dose limiting side effects

| | | | |
|---|---|---|---|
| Methacholine (Mecholyl) | Ampules: 25 mg | 0.1-0.4 mg/kg SC or IM as single dose; may increase by 25% q30 min. | Contraindicated in asthma, intestinal or bladder neck obstruction. May cause cholinergic crisis. Keep atropine available. |
| Methenamine Mandelate (Mandelamine) | Tablets: 250, 500, 1000 mg Susp: 500 mg/5 ml | Initial Dose: 100 mg/kg/day PO divided q8h Maintenance Dose: 50 mg/kg/day PO divided q8h (Max. total dose = 3 gm/day) | Contraindicated in renal insufficiency. Maintain urine acidity below pH 5.5. |
| Methicillin (Staphcillin) | Vials: 1 gm | 100-400 mg/kg/day IM or IV divided q4-6h Newborn: 100-200 mg/kg/day IM or IV divided q8-12h (Max. adult dose = 12 gm/day) | Allergic cross-reactivity with and same toxicity as penicillin. May cause hematuria and nephritis. |
| Methimazole (Tapazole) | Tablets: 5 + 10 mg | Initial: 0.4 mg/kg/day PO divided q8h Maintenance: 0.2 mg/kg/day PO divided q8h (average dose) | May cause blood dyscrasias, dermatitis, hepatitis, CNS reactions, arthralgia, or hypothyroidism. Follow thyroid function. 10 mg Tapazole = 100 mg PTU. |

157

| Methocarbamol (Robaxin) | Tablets: 500 mg<br>Ampules: 100 mg/ml | 15 mg/kg/dose PO, IM or IV q6h PRN (Max. single dose = 1 gm IM or IV) (Max. IV dosage rate in adults 300 mg/min. or 3 ml/min.) | Dose may be increased in treating tetanus. Avoid extravasation. May cause hypotension. |
| Methotrexate (Amethopterin) | Tablets: 2.5 mg<br>Vials: 5 + 50 mg | PO, IV, IT | Oral and G.I. ulcerations, diarrhea, hepatotoxic, pneumonitis *Bone marrow depression toxicity increased with renal dysfunction *Arachnoiditis, transverse myelitis and seizures reported with IT administration. |
| Methsuximide (Celontin) | Capsules: 150 + 300 mg<br>Susp: 300 mg/5 ml | Initial: 300 mg/day PO single dose<br>Increase: 300 mg/day increments/week PRN (Max. total dose = 1.2 gm) | May cause blood dyscrasias, GI, CNS symptoms, and behavioral changes. |
| Methylodopa (Aldomet) | Tablets: 250 mg<br>Ampules: 50 mg/ml | Oral: 10 mg/kg/day PO divided q8-12h; increase PRN at 2 day intervals<br>Intravenous (crisis): 20-40 mg/kg/day IV divided q6h (Max. total dose = 65 mg/kg/day) | Contraindicated in pheochromocytoma and active hepatic disease. False-positive Coomb's, fever, hemolytic anemia, leukopenia--follow liver function and hematologic status. |

*Dose limiting side effects

| | | | |
|---|---|---|---|
| Methylene Blue | Ampules: 10 mg/ml (1%) | Methemoglobinemia:<br>1-2 mg/kg/dose IV over<br>5 minutes. | |
| Methylphenidate<br>(Ritalin) | Tablets: 5 + 10 mg | Hyperactivity: 0.25-2 mg/kg/day PO divided into 2 or 3 doses | Contraindicated in epilepsy and glaucoma. May interact with pressors. |
| Metronidazole<br>(Flagyl) | Tablets: 250 mg<br>Vag. Supp: 500 mg | Trichimonas vaginalis<br>Orally: 250 mg q8h x 10 days (treat sexual partner with 250 mg q12h)<br>Vaginally: 500 mg supp. qd x 10 days<br>Giardiasis: 250 mg q6h x 10 days PO | Nausea, diarrhea, leukopenia. |
| Minocycline<br>(Minocin) | Capsules: 50 + 100 mg<br>Syrup: 50 mg/5 ml<br>Vial: 100 mg | Alternate drug for carriers of Sulfa-resistant meningococci:<br>Initial: 4 mg/kg x 1 dose<br>Then: 2 mg/kg q12h x 5 doses | High incidence of vestibular dysfunction. See Tetracycline. |

| Drug | Preparation | Dosage | Side Effects/Notes |
|---|---|---|---|
| Mithramycin (Mithracin) | Vials: 2500 microgram (refrigerate) | IV<br>Has been used in hypercalcemia associated with malignancies | Cellulitis on extravasation, nausea, vomiting, hypocalcemia, fever hepato and renal toxicity<br>*Bone marrow depression<br>*Hemorrhagic diathesis with coagulopathy. |
| Morphine | Vials: 8, 10, 15 mg/ml | Analgesia: 0.1-0.2 mg/kg/dose SC repeat q4h PRN<br>Tetralogy (cyanotic) Spells: 0.2 mg/kg/dose SC repeat q4h PRN (Max. total dose = 15 mg/dose) | For respiratory depression secondary to morphine overdose see Naloxone or Nalorphine. |
| Nafcillin (Unipen) | Capsule: 250 mg<br>Vials: 250 mg/ml | Newborn: 40 mg/day PO divided q6h; 20-40 mg/kg day IM divided q12h<br>Older Infants & Children: 50-100 mg/kg/day PO divided q6h; 100-200 mg/kg/day IM divided q12h, or IV q4h (Max. adult dose = 12 gm/day) | Allergic cross-sensitivity with penicillin. |
| Nalorphine (Nalline) | Ampules: 0.2 + 5 mg/ml | 0.1 mg/kg/dose IV or IM repeat q15 minutes PRN | Will cause increased CNS and respiratory depression if primary depression not due to narcotic. |

*Dose limiting side effects

| Drug | Form | Dosage | Comments |
|---|---|---|---|
| Naloxone (Narcan) | Ampules: 0.4 mg/ml (400 micrograms/ml) | 5-10 micrograms/kg/dose IM or IV repeat q2-3 minutes PRN x 3 | No respiratory depression. Experience in infants and children limited. |
| Neomycin Sulfate | Tablets: 500 mg Vials: 500 mg | Prematures & Newborns: 50 mg/kg/day PO divided q6h; Infants & Children: 100 mg/kg/day PO divided q6h | Contraindicated in intestinal obstruction and ulcerative bowel disease. Follow for signs of renal or oto-toxicity. |
| Neomycin + Polymixin B + Gramicidin (Neosporin) | Ophth. Soln: 10cc + droppers | 1-2 drops q6-12h | |
| Neostigmine (Prostigmin) | Tablets: 15 mg Ampules: 0.25 + 0.5 mg/ml Vials: 1 mg/ml | 2 mg/kg/day PO divided q3-4h; Myasthenia Gravis Test: 0.04 mg/kg/dose IM; 0.02 mg/kg/dose IV | Contraindicated in intestinal and urinary obstruction. May cause cholinergic crisis. Keep atropine available. |
| Niclosamide (Yomesan) | Tablets: 500 mg | <2 yr. 500 mg qd x 5 da; 2-8 yr. 1000 mg qd x 5 da; >8 yr. 2000 mg qd x 5 da | Drug of choice for tapeworms. Available from C.D.C., Parasitic Disease Branch Atlanta, Ga. 30333 |

| Drug | Preparation | Dosage | Side Effects |
|---|---|---|---|
| Nitrofurantoin (Furadantin) | Tablets: 50 + 100 mg Susp: 25 mg/5 ml | 5-7 mg/kg/day PO divided q6h (Max. adult dose = 400 mg/day) | Dosage may require reduction in prolonged use (>2 weeks). Contraindicated in severe renal disease, G6PD deficiency, and in infants <1 mo. of age. |
| Nitrogen Mustard | Vials: 10 mg powder with 10cc sterile water | IV | Cellulitis with extravasation, nausea, vomiting, alopecia, hypersensitivity rash, CNS toxicity, *Bone marrow depression. |
| Nystatin (Mycostatin) | Tablets: 500,000 units Susp: 100,000 units/ml Topical powder, cream, ointment, vaginal suppository: 100,000 units/gm | Premature & Newborn Infants: 400,000 units/day PO divided q6-8h Older Infants & Children: 1-2 million units/day PO divided q6-8h Vaginal: 1 supp qhs x 10 days | May produce diarrhea or GI symptoms. |
| Oral Citrate Mixture (Polycitra) | Syrup: 1 ml contains 2 mEq citrate, 1 mEq Na, and 1 mEq K. | 5-20 ml/dose PO q6-8h | Adjust dosage to maintain desired urine pH. |

*Dose limiting side effects

162

| Drug | Preparation | Dosage | Comments |
|---|---|---|---|
| PAS, p-amino-salicylic acid (Pamisyl) | Resin: 50% (acid) Powder: (Na salt) Tablets: (Ca + Na + K salts) Tablets, enteric coated: 500 mg (acid) | 300 mg/kg/day PO divided q8h (Max. total dose = 12 gm/day) | May cause hepatic damage, GI symptoms, renal damage, and hypothyroidism. 1 gm Na salt = 109 mg Na |
| Pancuronium Bromide (Pavulon) | Vials: 2 mg/ml | Neonates initial dose: 0.02 mg/kg/dose Older Children initial dose: 0.1-0.15 mg/kg. Use 0.01 mg/kg/dose for maintenance--must be given usually q30-40 min. | Must be prepared to intubate within 2 minutes of induction. Drug affect accentuated by halothane, diethyl ether, succinylcholine, hypokalemia and following broad spectrum antibiotics, i.e. neomycin, streptomycin, gentamycin, kanamycin and bacitracin. |
| Paraldehyde | Ampules: 1 gm/ml (5 ml) Oral Solution: 1 gm/ml (5 ml) | Sedative: 0.15 ml (150 mg)/kg/dose PO, IM, or PR in equal amount of oil Anticonvulsant: 0.15 ml (150 mg)/kg/dose q4-6h deep IM. 0.3 ml (300 mg)/kg/dose PR in oil q4-6h; 10 ml (10 gm) diluted in 90 cc normal saline & titrate 5-40 drops/min. (Max. dose = 8 ml) See Anticonvulsant section. | Do not use discolored solution. Avoid plastic syringes (use glass-it dissolves plastic). Contra-indicated in hepatic or pulmonary disease. Overdose may cause cardiorespiratory depression. IM may give sterile abscesses. |

| | | |
|---|---|---|
| Paregoric (Camphorated Opium Tincture) | Tinctures: 2 mg/5 ml (0.4 mg morphine/ml) | Narcotic withdrawal newborn: 2-4 drops/kg q4-6h may increase to 20-40 drops/kg/day Sedation: begin at 0.06 ml/month up to 12 months q3-4h (Max. dosage = 0.25-0.5 ml/kg/dose) | Same side effects as morphine. |
| Penicillamine (Cuprimine) | Capsules: 250 mg | Infants <6 mos.: 250 mg PO single daily dose Older Infants and Children: 1 gm/day PO divided q6h. Increase gradually based on clinical response and heavy metal excretion (Max. dose = 4-5 gm/day) | May cause blood dyscrasias, nephrotic syndrome, liver and skin disorders, cataracts and optic neuritis. |

| Penicillin G | Potassium salt: (Pen-Tids)<br>Tablets: 200,000 + 400,000 units<br>Oral Liquid: 200,000 + 400,000 units/5 ml<br>Vials: 1, 5, + 20 million units<br>Sodium Salt:<br>Vials: 1 + 5 million<br>Benzathine: (Bicillin)<br>Tablets: 200,000 units<br>Vials: 300,000 + 600,000 units/ml<br>Procaine: (Crysticillin, Duracillin):<br>Vials (aqueous):<br>500,000 units/ml | Na + K Salts:<br>Premature & Newborn:<br>30,000-150,000 units q8-12h<br>Full Term: 50,000-200,000 units q8-12h<br>Children: 25,000-300,000 units/kg/day PO, IM, or IV divided q4-6h<br>Benzathine 0.3-1.2 million units/dose IM. Do not use in newborns.<br>Procaine: 0.3-1.2 million units/day IM single daily dose. Do not use in newborns.<br>Rheumatic Fever Prophylaxis: 400,000 units/day PO divided q12h OR 1.2 million units Benzathine IM once monthly. | K Salt: 1 mg = 1,595 units. 1 million units contains 1.68 mEq (65.8 mg) K+<br>Na salt: 1 mg = 1,667 units. 1 million units contains 1.68 mEq (38.7 mg) Na+<br>Benzathine: 1 mg = 1,211 units<br>Procaine: 1 mg = 1,009 units. |

165

| | | |
|---|---|---|
| Penicillin V | Phenoxymethyl Penicillin: <br> Capsules: (V-Cillin) <br> 250 mg (400,000 units) <br> Tablets: (Pen Vee) <br> 125 + 300 mg <br> (200,000 + 500,000 units) <br> Phenoxymethyl Penicillin Potassium: <br> (Pen Vee K, V-Cillin K) <br> Tablets: 125 + 250 mg <br> (200,000 + 400,000 units) <br> Oral Solution: 125 + 250 mg/5 ml | Children: 25,000-50,000 units/kg/day PO divided q6h <br> Rheumatic Fever Prophylaxis: 250 mg (400,000 units)/day PO divided q12h | Phenoxymethyl: <br> 1 mg = 1,695 units <br> K Salt: <br> 1 mg = 1,530 units |
| Pentamidine Isethionate (Lomidine) | 100 mg/1cc (sterile water only) | 4 mg/kg/dose qd IM x 10 days for T. gambiense; x 12-14 days for Pneumocystis carinii. (Max. total dose = 56 mg/.kg) | Transient hypotension, tachycardia, nausea, vomiting, hypoglycemia, hypocalcemia, mild hepatotoxicity, mild anemia (megoloblastic) and granulocytopenia, renal toxocity-- available from CDC., Parasitic Dis. Branch, Atlanta, Ga. 30333 |

| | | | |
|---|---|---|---|
| Pentobarbital (Nembutal) | Capsules: 30, 50, 100 mg<br>Elixir: 20 mg/5 ml<br>Supp: 30, 60, 120, 200 mg<br>Ampules: 50 mg/ml<br>Vials: 50 mg/ml | Sedation: 2-3 mg/kg/dose PO, IM, or PR; repeat q8h PRN | No advantage over phenobarbital for control of convulsions. |
| Phenazopyridine (Pyridium) | Tablets: 100 mg | 12 mg/kg/day PO divided q8h | Use caution in presence of G6PD deficiency, GI problems or renal insufficiency. May cause methemoglobinemia. |
| Phenobarbital (Luminal) | Tablets: 15,30, 65 + 100 mg<br>Elixir: 20 mg/5 ml<br>Spansule: 60 + 100 mg<br>Vials: 65 mg/ml | Sedation: 2-3 mg/kg/dose PO, IM, or PR; repeat PRN q8h<br>Status Epilepticus: 10-15 mg total/kg IM or preferably slowly IV with caution. Give 1/2 above dose stat then 1/4 dose q5 min. x 2 or until seizure stops<br>Chronic Anticonvulsant: 4-6 mg/kg/day PO divided q12h is the average starting dose | IV administration may cause respiratory arrest or hypotension. Contraindicated in hepatic or renal disease and porphyria. |

| Drug | Preparation | Dosage | Comments |
|---|---|---|---|
| Phentolamine (Regitine) | Vials: 5 mg/ml | Pheochromocytoma Test: 0.1 mg/kg IV single dose Therapeutic: 5 mg/kg/day PO divided q4-6h | May cause hypotension, arrhythmias, and GI disturbances. |
| Phenylephrine (Neo-Syn-ephrine) | Vials: 10 mg/ml (1% solution) Nasal Solution: 0.25, 0.5, 1.0% Ophthalmic Solution: 10% | 0.1 mg/kg/dose SC or IM q1-2h PRN 1.0 mg/kg/day PO divided q4h IV Infusion: 10 mg/100 ml saline - adjust dosage rate to desired effect. See anti-arrhythmic drugs | Use with caution in presence of hypertension, arrhythmias, hyperthyroidism, or hyperglycemia. |
| Pilocarpine Hydrochloride (Pilocar) | Ophthalmic solution: 1, 2, 3, 4, 6, 8% | 1 or 2 drops O.U. PRN | |
| Piperazine (Antepar) | Tablets: 500 mg Syrup: 500 mg/ml | Enterobiasis + Oxyuriasis: 50 mg/kg/day PO single daily dose x 7 days Ascariasis: 50-75 mg/kg/day PO single daily dose x 2 days (Max. dose = 4 gm/day) | Contraindicated in epilepsy. Large doses may cause vomiting, urticaria, muscle weakness, blurred vision. |

| Polymyxin B (Aerosporin) | Vials: 50 mg (1 mg = 10,000 units) Otic Soln: 1 mg/ml | Enteric: 10-20 mg/kg/day PO divided q6h Systemic: Prematures & Newborns: 2.5-4.0 mg/kg/day divided q6h IM or q12h IV. Older Children: 2.5-3.0 mg/kg/day divided q4-6h IM or 1.5-2.5 mg/kg/day divided q12h IV (Max. dose = 200 mg/day) Intrathecal or Intraventricular: <2 yrs: 1-2 mg/day as single daily dose x 3-4 doses then qod. >2 yrs: 2.5-5.0 mg/day as single daily dose x 3-4 days then qod. | IV Route: Give by slow infusion over 1-2 hours IM Route: Difficult in older children because of severe pain. Pervasive renal and neurotoxocity. Does not cross blood-brain barrier. |
| Potassium Iodide (SSKI) | Tablets: 300 mg Solution: 100% | Expectorant: 2-4 drops in orange juice PO q8h Thyrotoxicosis: 0.9 ml or 900 mg KI/day PO divided q8h | Contraindicated in tuberculosis. |

169

| Potassium Supplements | Potassium Chloride: (1.0 gm salt = 13.3 mEq K) Tablets (enteric coated): 0.3 + 1.0 gm Oral Solution and Oral Syrup (wild cherry): 500 mg/5 ml (10%) Potassium Gluconate: (Kaon) (1.0 gm salt = 4.3 mEq K) Elixir: 1.56 gm/5 ml 6.66 mEq K/5 ml) Potassium Triplex: (Acetate-bicarbonate-citrate) Oral Solution: 500 mg of each salt/5 ml (15 mEq K/5 ml) | Dose based upon clinical requirements. | May cause GI disturbances and ulceration. Avoid overdosage. |
| Primidone (Mysoline) | Tablets: 50 + 250 mg Susp: 250 mg/5 ml | Initial: <8 yrs: 125 mg/day PO as single dose x 1 week. >8 yrs: 250 mg/day PO as single dose x 1 week. Increase: Weekly increments of 125-250 mg (Max. = 2 gm/day) to desired effect. Divided q12h PO. | May cause megaloblastic anemia, hallucinations and other emotional reactions, CNS disturbances, rashes, and GI symptoms. Do not discontinued abruptly. |

| Drug | Forms | Dosage | Toxicity |
|---|---|---|---|
| Procainamide (Pronestyl) | Capsules: 250 mg<br>Vials: 100 mg/ml (10 ml) | PO: 40-60 mg/kg/day divided q4-6h<br>IM: 20-30 mg/kg/day divided q6h<br>IV: 2 mg/kg/dose (Max. dose = 100 mg) diluted and given by slow infusion over 5 minutes repeat q10-30 minutes PRN. (Max. total daily dose = 2-4 gm PO or IM or 1-2 gm IV) | Monitor BP and EKG with IV use. Widening of QRS by more than 0.02 seconds suggests toxicity (stop or skip dose). |
| Procarbazine (Matulane) | Capsules: 50 mg | PO | Nausea, vomiting, lethargy, CNS depression, alopecia, stomatitis neuropathy, *Bone marrow depression. |
| Prochlorperazine (Compazine) | Tablets: 5 mg<br>Syrup: 5 mg/5 ml<br>Supp: 5 + 25 mg<br>Spansule: 10 + 15 mg<br>Ampules: 5 mg/ml | 0.4 mg/kg/day PO or PR divided q6-8h<br>0.2 mg/kg/day IM divided q6-8h | Toxicity as for other phenothiazines. CNS reactions not uncommon (extrapyramidal). |

*Dose limiting side effects

| | | | |
|---|---|---|---|
| Promethazine (Phenergan) | Tablets: 12.5 + 25 mg<br>Ampules: 25 mg/ml | Antihistaminic:<br>0.1 mg/kg/dose q6h and 0.5 mg/kg/dose hs PO PRN<br>Nausea and Vomiting:<br>0.25-0.5 mg/kg/dose IM or PR q4-6h PRN<br>Sedative & Preoperative:<br>0.5-1.0 mg/kg/dose IM q6h PRN<br>Motion Sickness:<br>0.5 mg/kg/dose PO q12h PRN | Toxicity similar to other phenothiazines. (See Chlorpromazine.) |
| Propantheline (Pro-Banthine) | Tablets: 15 mg<br>Vials: 30 mg | 1-2 mg/kg/day PO divided qid pc and hs | Contraindicated in glaucoma and cardiac disease. |
| Propoxyphene (Darvon) | Capsules: 32 + 65 mg | 2-3 mg/kg/day PO divided q4-6h | |

| Drug | Form | Dosage | Comments |
|---|---|---|---|
| Propranolol (Inderal) | Tablets: 10 + 40 mg<br>Ampules: 1 mg/ml | **Arrhythmias:**<br>0.01-0.15 mg/kg/dose, slow IV push may repeat q6-8h PRN (Max. single dose = 10 mg).<br>0.5-1.0 mg/kg/day PO divided q6-8h (Max. daily dose = 60 mg).<br>**Tetralogy spells:** 0.15-0.25 mg/kg/dose IV slowly --may repeat in 15 min. x 1 (Max single dose = 10 mg)<br>Maintenance: 1-2 mg/kg/dose q6h PO<br>**Thyrotoxicosis:** PO 2.5-10.5 mg/kg/dose q6-8h (average dose 3.5 mg/kg/dose). Start at lower dose and increase slowly q2h until effective.<br>IV Adult Dose: 1-2 mg IV push slowly over 10 min. | Contraindicated in asthma and heart block. Use with caution in presence of obstructive lung disease, heart failure, renal or hepatic disease. May cause hypoglycemia, hypotension, nausea, vomiting. |
| Propyl-thiouracil (PTU) | Tablets: 50 mg | **Initial:** 6-10 yrs: 150-300 mg/day PO >10 yrs: 300-400 mg/day PO<br>**Maintenance:** (When euthyroid) 75-200 mg/day PO divided q8-12h | May cause blood dyscrasias, fever, liver disease, and dermatitis. Monitor thyroid function. 100 mg PTU = 10 mg Tapazole. |

| Protamine | Ampules: 10 mg/ml | Heparin Antidote: 1 mg for every 1 mg heparin in previous 3-4h by IV drip (Max. dose = 50 mg/dose) | May cause coagulation problem in absence of heparin. (120 units heparin = 1 mg.) |
|---|---|---|---|
| Pseudoephedrine (Sudafed) | Tablets: 60 mg Syrup: 30 mg/5 ml | 4-5 mg/kg/day PO divided q6h | Use with caution in hypertension. |
| Pyrantel (Antiminth) | Susp: 50 mg/ml | Ascaris and pinworms: 10 mg/kg/dose (single dose) PO | Nausea, vomiting, transient SGOT elevations. |
| Pyrivinium (Povan) | Tablets: 50 mg Susp: 50 mg/5 ml | 5 mg/kg/dose PO as single dose; repeat in 2 weeks | May cause GI symptoms. Colors stools red. |
| Quinacrine (Atabrine) | Tablets: 100 mg | Giardiasis: 8 mg/kg/day PO q8h. Give single dose 1st day, 2 doses 2nd day, and full 8 mg/kg/day in 3 doses 3rd day x 5 days. (Max. dose = 300 mg/day) Tapeworms: 15 mg/kg/day PO divided into 2 doses 1 hour apart. Saline purge 2 hours after last dose and night before first dose. (Max. dose = 800 mg) | May cause GI disturbances. |

| Drug | Preparations | Dosage | Remarks |
|---|---|---|---|
| Quinidine | Gluconate:<br>Tablets: 330 mg<br>Vials: 80 mg/ml<br>Sulfate:<br>Tablets: 200 mg<br>Extended Release<br>Tablets: 300 mg | Test dose: 2 mg/kg/dose PO<br>Therapeutic dose:<br>Sulfate: 3-6 mg/kg/dose<br>PO repeated q2-3h x 5<br>Gluconate: 2-10 mg/kg/<br>dose IV repeat q3-6h PRN | Toxicity indicated by increase of QRS interval by 0.02 seconds or more (skip dose or stop drug). May cause GI symptoms, hypotension, tinnitus, blood dyscrasias. |
| Reserpine (Serpasil) | Tablets: 0.1 + 0.25 mg<br>Ampules: 2.5 mg/ml<br>Vials: 2.5 mg/ml | General Use & Chronic Hypertension: 0.02 mg/kg/day PO divided q12h<br>Acute Hypertension: 0.07 mg/kg/dose IM repeat q8-24 hours PRN (use with hydralazine if necessary.) Due to hypersensitivity (marked hypotension) of some patients, 1/10 of dose should be given initially IM. (Max. dose 2.5 mg/day)<br>Ref: PCNA 21:818, 1974 | May cause CNS and respiratory depression in newborns of treated mothers. Discontinue 2 or more weeks before elective surgery. |
| Rifampin (Rimactane) | Capsules: 300 mg<br>Syrup: 20 mg/ml | Antituberculosis:<br>10-20 mg/kg/day PO as single dose (Max. dose = 600 mg/day)<br>Sulfa Resistant Meningococci Carriers:<br>10 mg/kg/dose q12h x 2 da | Use with caution in liver dysfunction. Not officially released yet for children. |

| | | |
|---|---|---|
| Salicylazo-sulfapyridine (Azulfidine) | Tablets: 500 mg | Initial: 75-150 mg/kg/day PO divided q4-8h Maintenance: 40 mg/kg/day PO divided q6h (Max. adult dose = 6 gm/day) | See Sulfisoxazole. |
| Scopolamine (Hyoscine) | Tablets: 400 + 600 micrograms Vials: 1 milligram /ml | 6 micrograms/kg/dose PO or SC | See Atropine. |
| Secobarbital (Seconal) | Capsules: 32, 50, 100 mg Supp: 60 mg Vials: 50 mg/ml | Sedation: 6 mg/kg/day PO divided q8h | See Amobarbital. |
| Sodium Polystyrene Sulfonate (Kayexalate) | Oral Powder: 450 gm Susp: 25%, in sorbitol solution (25%) | Practical Exchange Rate: 1 mEq potassium per 1 gm resin. Calculate dose according to desired exchange. PO or rectally q6h PRN | Use with caution in presence of renal failure. (Na+ exchanged for K+; may also cause hypocalcemia and hypomagnesemia.) |
| Spironolactone (Aldactone) | Tablets: 25 mg | 1.7-3.3 mg/kg/day PO divided q6-8h | Contraindicated in acute renal insufficiency. May potentiate ganglionic blocking agents and other antihypertensives. May cause hyperkalemia. |

| | | | |
|---|---|---|---|
| Streptomycin | Vials: 400 mg/ml | Premature & Full term<br>Newborn: 15-25 mg/kg/day IM divided q12h up to 10 days.<br>Children: 40 mg/kg/day IM divided q8h up to 10 days<br>Tuberculosis: 20-50 mg/kg/day IM single dose (use higher dose for TB meningitis)<br>(Max. dose = 2 gm/day) | Reduce dose in presence of renal insufficiency. Follow auditory status. May cause CNS depression and other neurologic manifestations. |
| Succinyl-choline (Anectine) | Vials: 20 mg/ml | 1-2 mg/kg initial dose IV. Duration of action 10 min. Prolonged relaxation should be controlled by intermittent IV infusion of 0.5-1 mg/kg. Titrate according to response. | Must be able to intubate patient within 1 minute. Side effects include bradycardia, hypotension, arrhythmia. Beware of prolonged depression in patients with pseudocholin-esterase deficiency. |
| Sulfacetamide Sodium (Sulamyd) | Ophth Soln: 10%, 15%, 30%<br>Ophth Oint: 10% | Apply q3-4h | See Sulfisoxazole. |

| | | | |
|---|---|---|---|
| Sulfadiazine | Tablets: 500 mg<br>Susp: 500 mg/5 ml<br>Ampules: 250 mg/ml | See Sulfisoxazole. | See Sulfisoxazole. |
| Sulfathiazole<br>+ Sulfabenza-<br>mide +<br>Sulfacetamide<br>(Sultrin) | Vaginal Cream and<br>Tablets | Apply cream BID x 4-6 days<br>or 1 tablet qd x 10 days | See Sulfisoxazole. |
| Sulfisoxazole<br>(Gantrisin) | Tablets: 500 mg<br>Susp: 500 mg/5 ml<br>Ampules: 400 mg/ml<br>Ophth Soln: 40 mg/ml<br>Ophth Oint: 40 mg/gm | Initial: 75 mg/kg/dose PO;<br>50 mg/kg/dose IV<br>Maintenance: 150 mg/kg/day<br>PO divided q4-6h; 100 mg/<br>kg/day IV divided q6h<br>(Max. dose = 8 gm/day)<br>Rheumatic Fever Prophyla-<br>xis: <30 kg: 500 mg/day/<br>PO single dose. >30 kg:<br>1 gm/day PO single dose.<br>Ophth Soln: 2-3 drops<br>q4-8h<br>Ophth Oint: 1-3 times<br>daily | Contraindicated in in-<br>fants under 2 months,<br>near-term pregnant or<br>nursing mothers. Use<br>with caution in pre-<br>sence of renal or liver<br>disease, or G6PD defi-<br>ciency. Maintain ade-<br>quate fluid intake. |

178

| | Preparations | Dose | Dose determined by theophylline content |
|---|---|---|---|
| Tedral | Tablets:<br>Theophylline 130 mg<br>Ephedrine 24 mg<br>Phenobarbital 8 mg<br>(per tablet)<br>Pediatric Susp:<br>Theophylline 65 mg<br>Ephedrine 12 mg<br>Phenobarbital 4 mg<br>(per 5 ml) | Pediatric Suspension:<br>5 ml/30 kg/dose repeat q6h PRN | Dose determined by theophylline content |
| Tetracycline (Achromycin) | Tablets: 50, 100, 250 mg<br>Capsules: 50, 100, 250 mg<br>Drops: 100 mg/ml<br>Syrup: 25 mg/ml<br>Susp: 50 mg/ml<br>Vials: 100,250, 500 mg | Older Infants & Children<br>25-50 mg/kg/day PO divided q6h<br>10-25 mg/kg/day IM divided q8-12h<br>10-15 mg/kg/day IV divided q12h<br>Children >40 kg:<br>1-2 gm/day PO divided q6h<br>10-20 mg/kg/day IM or IV divided q12h (Max. dose = 2 gm/day) | RECOMMENDED ONLY WHEN ANOTHER DRUG IS NOT SUITABLE. May cause increased intracranial pressure, tooth staining, decreased bone growth, and GI reactions. Outdated drug may cause nephropathy. Not recommended in newborns and infants. |
| Theophylline (Elixophyllin) | Elixir: 27 mg/5 ml<br>Capsule: 200 mg | 5-10 mg/kg/dose q6h.<br>Start at lower dose and increase q3 days<br><br>Ref: J. Ped. 84:421, 1974 | Use with caution in cardiac, renal, hepatic hyperthyroid, ulcer disease and glaucoma (See Aminophylline). Most common side effect vomiting. |

| | | | |
|---|---|---|---|
| Thiabendazole (Mintezol) | Susp: 500 mg/ml | 25 mg/kg/dose PO bid PC. Threadworms, Hookworms, Ascaris: 1-2 days Whipworms: 2-4 days Pinworms: 1 day, repeat in 1 week | Caution in hepatic disease. May cause GI symptoms and dizziness. |
| 6-Thioguanine | Tablet: 40 mg | PO | Nausea, vomiting, *Bone marrow depression |
| Thyroid (desiccated) | Tablets: 15, 30, 60, 130, 180 mg | Initial: Infants: 15 mg/dose PO single daily dose Children: 30 mg/dose PO single daily dose Usual Maintenance: 60-180 mg/day PO single daily dose. Increase by 15 mg/day at weekly intervals. | Follow and titrate with serum T4 level. |
| Tolnaftate (Tinactin) | Cream: 1% Solution: 1% Powder: 1% | Apply cream or 1 or 2 gtts of solution topically bid for 2 to 6 weeks | Persistent infection may require systemic therapy with griseofulvin. |

*Dose limiting side effects

| Drug | Preparations | Dosage | Comments |
|---|---|---|---|
| Triiodothyronine (Cytomel) | Tablets: 5 + 25 micrograms | Calculate dosage as for desicated thyroid according to following equivalencies: 65 mg (1 grain) USP desicated thyroid = 25 micrograms triiodothyronine | See Thyroid. |
| Trimethadone (Tridione) | Capsules: 300 mg | Initial dose: 20-50 mg/kg/day q6-8h PO Increase by: 150-300 mg increments to desired clinical effect or toxicity | Contraindicated in severe hepatic or renal disease or blood dyscrasias. May cause lupus-like symptoms and nephrosis. |
| Trimethobenzamide (Tigan) | Capsules: 100 + 250 mg Supp: 100 + 200 mg Ampules: 100 mg/ml | 15 mg/kg/day PO, PR, or IM divided q6-8h PRN | IM route not recommended for infants. |
| Trimethoprim-Sulfamethoxazole (Spectra) (Bactrim) | Tablets: 80 mg trimethoprim 400 mg sulfamethoxazole | Trimethoprim: 8-10 mg/kg/day PO q6h Sulfamethoxazole: 40-50 mg/kg/day PO q6h | See sulfisoxazole. Not released for <12 yr. old. |

| | | | |
|---|---|---|---|
| Tripelennamine (Pyribenzamine) | Tablets: 25 + 50 mg Long-acting tablets: 100 mg Elixir: 37.5 mg/5 ml | 5 mg/kg/day PO divided q4-6h (Max. dose = 300 mg/day) | |
| Tromethamine (Tris, Tham) | 0.3 M soln. | Total Dose 0.3M Tham (ml) = kg of body weight x base deficit. 1/4 dose over 2-5 min; 1/4 dose slowly over 3-6 hrs; additional dose according to degree of acidosis. Total 24 hr. should not exceed 33-40 ml/kg<br><br>Ref: Ped 41:667, 1968 Pediatric Therapy, 4th edition, 228-261. | Must monitor blood pH, pCO2, pO2 hourly. Do not attempt to buffer blood pH>7.25-7.30. Side effects include hypoglycemia, hyperkalemia, osmotic diuresis. Do not use in renal failure. Beware tissue necrosis and extravasation. |
| Vasopressin (Pitressin) | Ampules: 20 units/ml (aqueous) Ampules: 5 units/ml (tannate in oil) Nose drops: 50 units/ml (arginine vasopressin - Diapid) | Aqueous: 1-3 ml/day SC divided q8h. Tannate in Oil: 0.2 ml/ dose IM q1-3 day PRN; may increase to 1-2 ml/ dose Nose drops: 1-2 gtts qhs each nostril q4-6h PRN | |

| Vinblastine (Velban) | Vials: 10 mg (refrigerate) | IV | Cellulitis on extravasation, nausea, vomiting, stomatitis, alopecia, areflexia, *Bone marrow depression |
|---|---|---|---|
| Vincristine (Oncovin) | Vials: 1 + 5 mg (refrigerate) | IV | Cellulitis on extravasation, peripheral neuropathy, areflexia, alopecia, abdominal pain with paralytic ileus, jaw pain, constipation. *Bone marrow depression, *Neurotoxicity |
| Vitamin K (Aqua-Mephyton) (Konakion) | Tablets: 5 mg Ampules: 1 mg/ml (Aqueous) Ampules: 10 mg/ml (emulsion) | Hemorrhagic Disease of Newborn: Prophylaxis: 1 mg IM Treatment: 5-10 mg IM Hypoprothrombinemia: Infants: 2 mg/dose PO, IM, IV Children: 5-10 mg/dose PO, IM, IV | Follow protime. Use with caution in presence of severe hepatic disease. Large doses (>25 mg) in newborn may cause hyperbilirubinemia. |

*Dose limiting side effects

CARDIAC RESUSCITATION DRUGS

| | STOCK SOLUTION | DILUTION | FINAL CONCENTRATION | IV DOSAGE | RATE |
|---|---|---|---|---|---|
| Epinephrine | 1:1000 (1.0 mg/ml) | 1.0 ml in 9.0 ml/normal saline | 1:10,000 (0.1 mg/ml) | Newborn: 0.1 ml/kg Older: 1-5 ml | q3-5 min. |
| NaHCO3 (Sodium Bicarbonate) | 3.75 gm/50 ml (0.89 meq/ml) | | | Newborn: 2-4 meq/kg >15 kg: 50 ml (1 amp) | q10 min. |
| Isoproterenol (Isuprel) | 0.2 mg/ml (5 ml/vial) | 0.4 mg/100cc (one 5cc vial in 250cc) | 4 microgram/ml | 1-4 microgram/ min. | Continual IV perfusion |
| Calcium Chloride | 10% (100 mg/ml) | | | Newborn: 0.5-1.0 ml Older:increase to 10cc | q30-60 min. q3-5 min. (1-2 ml/min.) |

DIGITALIS AND ALLIED PREPARATIONS

| PREPARATION | EFFECT Earliest | EFFECT Max. | EFFECT Duration | TOTAL EXCRETION | ORAL ABSORPTION | ROUTE OF ADMINISTRATION | DOSE Digitalizing | DOSE Daily Maintenance |
|---|---|---|---|---|---|---|---|---|
| OUABAIN (G. Strophanthin) | 5 min. | 30 min. | 2 hrs. | 24-48 hours | 0 | IV only | TDD = 10 microgram/kg stat. 5 microgm/kg stat. 1 microgm/kg q 30 min. until response or total dose given. | Redigitalize with long-acting drug 12 hrs. after onset of Rx. |
| DIGIFOLINE | 2 hrs. | 4 hrs. | 2 days | 3 weeks | | IV OR IM | TDD = 25-30 microgram/kg 1/2 dose stat & 1/4 dose q6h x 2; or 1/6 dose stat and 1/6 dose q6h x 5. | 0.1 TDD |
| LANATOSIDE-C Cedilanid | 10-30 min. | 2 hrs. | 18-36 hrs. | 3-6 days | 10-20% | IV (best) or IM | TDD = 25 microgram/kg 1/2 dose stat; then 1/4 dose q2h x 2. | Use long-acting drug for maintenance. Redigitalize with long-acting drug after 24 hrs. |

DIGITALIS AND ALLIED PREPARATIONS (continued)

| PREPARATION | EFFECT | | | TOTAL EXCRE-TION | ORAL ABSORP-TION | ROUTE OF ADMINIS-TRATION | DOSE | |
|---|---|---|---|---|---|---|---|---|
| | Earli-est | Max. | Dura-tion | | | | Digitalizing | Daily Maintenance |
| DIGITOXIN Crystodigen Digisidin Digitaline Nativelle Purodigin | 30 min. | 6 hrs. | 2 days | 2-3 weeks | 100% | PO, IV, IM | TDD = 25-35 microgram/kg<br><br>1/2 dose stat, and 1/4 dose q6h x 2; or 1/6 dose stat and 1/6 dose q6h x 5. | 0.1-0.2 TDD |
| DIGOXIN (LANOXIN) 0.25 & 0.5 mg tablets 0.05 mg/ml elixir | 5-30 min. | 4-8 hrs. | 24 hrs. | 48-72 hrs. | 50-90*% consensus - 66% | PO, IM, IV | Premature & new born: TDD = 30-50 microgram/kg IM<br>Under age 2 yrs: TDD = 60-80 microgram/kg PO; 40-60 microgram/kg IM or IV<br>Over age 2 yrs: TDD = 40-60 microgm/kg PO; 20-40 microgm/kg IM or IV 1/2 dose stat; then 1/4 dose q6-8h x 2. | 0.25 TDD PO 0.20 TDD IM or IV divide q12h Usual adult maintenance 0.25-0.50/day. |

*Circ., 26:709, 1962.

186

INTRAVENOUS ANTI-ARRHYTHMIA DRUGS

| DRUG | DOSE | INDICATIONS | CAUTIONS |
|---|---|---|---|
| | | **TACHYARRHYTHMIAS** | |
| Digitalis Preparations | See page 184-185 | Supraventricular arrhythmias:<br>1) PAT or PNT unresponsive to vagal stimulation. Also PAT in Wolff-Parkinson-White Syndrome<br>2) Atrial flutter – fibrillation. | Contraindicated in ventricular arrhythmias. May cause heart block and other arrhythmias. Monitor EKG. |
| Diphenyl-hydantoin (Dilantin) | 1-5 mg/kg slow IV push repeat PRN (Max. total dose = 500 mg in 4 hrs.) | 1) Ventricular arrhythmias especially ventricular tachycardia.<br>2) Digitalis-induced arrhythmias, especially PAT with block. | Bradycardia. Monitor EKG. Hypertension. |
| Lidocaine (Xylocaine) | Slow IV Push: 2% solution: 0.5-1.0 mg/kg/ dose repeat q5-10 min. PRN.<br>Continuous IV Drip: 20-40 micrograms/kg/ min. (Max. total dose = 5 mg/kg) | Ventricular arrhythmias. | May cause hypotension, seizures, and cardiac or respiratory arrest. Monitor BP and EKG. |

187

INTRAVENOUS ANTI-ARRHYTHMIA DRUGS (continued)

| DRUG | DOSE | INDICATIONS | CAUTIONS |
|---|---|---|---|
| Metaraminol (Aramine) | 50 mg in 100cc D5W IV drip (Max. dose = 2 mg/kg) | PAT or PNT unresponsive to digitalis. | Titrate to desired effect. Pressor drug. Monitor BP and EKG. |
| Phenylephrine hydrochloride (Neo-syn-ephrine) | 10 mg (1 ml of 1% soln.) in 100 ml saline as continuous IV infusion. Titrate to desired effect. | PAT or PNT unresponsive to digitalis. | Pressor agent. May cause bradycardia and other arrhythmias. Monitor blood pressure and EKG. |
| Procainamide hydrochloride (Pronestyl) | 2 mg/kg/dose in D5W IV slowly over 5 min. Repeat q10-30 min. PRN (Max. dose = 100 mg) | Ventricular tachycardia and flutter. Supraventricular arrhythmias unresponsive to digitalis. | May produce ventricular arrhythmias and hypotension. Monitor BP and EKG. |
| Propranolol (Inderal) | General Arrhythmias: 0.01-0.15 mg/kg/dose slow IV push, may repeat q6-8h PRN (Max. single dose = 10 mg) Tetralogy Spells: 0.15-0.25 mg/kg/dose IV slowly, may repeat in 15 min. x 1 (Max. single dose = 10 mg) | Ventricular tachycardia, PVC's and digitalis-induced arrhythmias. Supraventricular tachycardia unresponsive to digitalis. Tetralogy spells. | May cause hypotension, hypoglycemia, bradycardia, and bronchospasm. Monitor BP and EKG. |

INTRAVENOUS ANTI-ARRHYTHMIA DRUGS (continued)

| DRUG | DOSE | INDICATIONS | CAUTIONS |
|------|------|-------------|----------|
| Quinidine gluconate | 2-10 mg/kg/dose IV repeat q3-6h PRN | Ventricular arrhythmias, atrial flutter or fibrillation, and to prevent PAT in Wolff-Parkinson-White Syndrome. | Use for atrial arrhythmias only in well-digitalized patient. May cause ventricular arrhythmias (increase in QRS by 0.02 or more) and hypotension. Monitor EKG and BP. |
| | | BRADYARRHYTHMIAS | |
| Atropine | 0.01-0.03 mg/kg/IV repeat PRN | | |
| Epinephrine | Intracardiac: 0.25-2.0 ml 1:1000 soln. IV: 4-8 mg/min. | | Ventricular ectopic beats--tachycardia. |
| Isoproterenol (Isuprel) | 1-4 mg/liter D5W as continuous IV infusion. Rate: 0.5-4.0 micrograms/minute. | Complete heart block or severe bradycardia. | Use care in presence of congestive failure or ventricular irritability. Monitor EKG. |

ACUTE ANTI-CONVULSANTS FOR STATUS EPILEPTICUS

| ANTICONVULSANT | DOSAGE AND ROUTE OF ADMINISTRATION | COMMENTS |
|---|---|---|
| Valium Ampules: 5 mg/ml | Intravenous diluted in sterile water, 0.5-0.75 mg/kg given slowly over minutes. Repeat x 2 every 15 min. Single dose not to exceed 10 mg. *Not good maintenance drug | Hypotension and respiratory depression particularly following barbiturates or paraldehyde. |
| Paraldehyde 1 gm/ml | Rectal: 0.3 ml/kg. Repeat 4-6 hourly. Deep intramuscular: 0.15 ml/kg repeat 4-6 hourly. (Adult max. 4-10 ml) Intravenous perfusion: 10 ml in 90 ml. normal saline titrated according to patients needs (5-40 drops/hr.) | Action delayed one-half hr. Sterile abscesses. Solution should not be allowed to stand in plastic bags. |
| Dilantin 20 mg/ml + 50 mg/ml | Loading dose: Intravenous perfusion 15 mg/kg in normal saline (50 mg/minute). Maintenance: 5-8 mg/kg once daily. Should not be given intramuscularly. | Monitor blood pressure and cardiac rate. |
| Phenobarbital 65 mg/ml | IM: 10 mg/kg IV: Give 5 mg/kg IV slowly then 2.5 mg/kg IV q 5 min. x 2 or until seizure stops. Chronic Anticonvulsant: 4-6 mg/kg/day PO q12h starting dose. | Monitor BP, respiration. DO NOT use with hepatic or renal disease, or porphyria. |

INSULIN

| | Dose determined by clinical situation | | | | | |
|---|---|---|---|---|---|---|
| Type of Insulin | Time and Route of Administration | Time of onset Hrs. after administration | Peak act- Hrs. after administration | Duration of Action Hrs. | Time when glycosuria most apt to occur | Time when hypoglycemia most apt to occur |
| *Crystalline Zinc | IV (emergency) 15-20 min. before meals, SC | Rapid--within 1 hour | 2-4 | 5-8 | During night | 10 a.m. to lunch |
| *Semi-Lente (Amorphous Zinc) | 1/2-3/4 hr. before breakfast; deep SC, never IV | Rapid--within 1 hour | 6-10 | 12-16 | During night | Before lunch |
| Globin Zinc | 1/2-1 hour before breakfast, SC | Intermediate-- rapidity of onset increases with dose, within 2-4 hours. | 6-10 | 18-24 also increases with dose. | Before breakfast & before lunch | 3 p.m. to dinner |
| *Lente (combination of 30% semi-lente & 70% ultra-lente) | 1 hour before breakfast; deep SC; never IV | Intermediate-- within 2-4 hrs. | 8-12 | 28-32 | Before lunch | 3 p.m. to dinner |
| NPH (Neutral-Protamine-Hagedorn) or Isophane | 1 hour before breakfast; SC | Intermediate-- within 2-4 hrs. | 8-12 | 28-30 | Before lunch | 3 p.m. to dinner |

*Contain no modifying protein, i.e., protamine or globin.

INSULIN (continued)

| Dose determined by clinical situation | | | | | | |
|---|---|---|---|---|---|---|
| Type of Insulin | Time and Route of Administration | Time of onset Hrs. after administration | Peak act- Hrs. after adminis- tration | Duration of Action Hrs. | Time when glyco- suria Most apt to occur | Time when hypo- glycemia most apt to occur |
| Protamine Zinc (PZI) | 1 hour before breakfast; SC | Slow-acting-- within 4-6 hrs | 16-24 | 24-36+ | Before lunch and at bedtime | 2 a.m. to breakfast |
| *Ultra-lente | 1 hour before breakfast; deep SC, never IV | Very slow-- 8 hours | 16-24 | 36+ | | During night, early morning |

*Contain no modifying protein, i.e., protamine or globin.

## ADRENAL GLUCOCORTICOIDS

HOW SUPPLIED:

Cortisone Acetate      Tablets: 5 + 25 mg
                          Vials:    25 + 50 mg/ml

Hydrocortisone:         Tablets: 5, 10 + 20 mg
                          Susp:    2 mg/ml
                          Vial:     5 mg/ml
     Na succinate: (Solu-Cortef)
                          Vials:    100, 250 + 500 mg
       Acetate:        Vials:    25 mg/ml

Prednisone:            Tablets: 1 + 5 mg

Prednisolone:          Tablets: 5 mg
                          Vials: 25 + 50 mg

Methylprednisolone:    Tablets: 4 mg
                          Extended Release Tablets: 4 mg
     Na succinate: (Solu-Medrol)
                          Vials:    40, 125 + 1000 mg
       Acetate:      (Depo-Medrol)
                          Vials:    40 mg/ml

Triamcinolone:          Tablets: 1, 2 + 4 mg
                          Vials:    10 + 40 mg/ml
                          Topical Cream: 0.025, 0.1, 0.5%
                          Topical Ointment: 0.01, 0.1%
                          Lotion:    0.025%

Dexamethasone:         Tablets: 0.5 + 0.75 mg
                          Oral Liquid: 0.5 mg/5 ml
                          Vials:     4 mg/ml
                          Cream:     0.1%

DOSE AND ROUTE:

Cortisone Acetate:

Physiologic Replacement:

25 mg/m$^2$/day PO divided q8h
12 mg/m$^2$/day IM single daily dose

Virilizing Adrenal Hyperplasia:

25 mg/m$^2$/day PO divided q8h
37 mg/m$^2$/dose IM every 3 days

ADRENAL GLUCOCORTICOIDS continued:

Prednisone:

Physiologic Replacement and General Use:

20% of cortisone dose

Therapeutic:

Leukemia and Lymphomas: 40-120 mg/m$^2$/day
PO divided q9-12h
Nephrotic Syndrome:* 2 mg/kg/day PO
single or divided doses
Rheumatic Carditis: 1.5-2.0 mg/kg/day PO
single or divided doses
Tuberculosis: 1-2 mg/kg/day PO single or
divided doses

Hydrocortisone sodium succinate:

Gram negative shock:

Initial dose:         50 mg/kg/IV
Subsequent dosage:    50-75 mg/kg/day IV
                      divided q6h
(Max. single dose = 500 mg)

Status Asthmaticus:   10 mg/kg/day IV
                      divided q6h

REMARKS:

Equivalent Doses For Same Clinical Effects

| DRUG | Glucocorticoid Anti-Inflammatory | Mineralo-corticoid |
|---|---|---|
| Cortisone acetate | 100 mg | 100 mg |
| Hydrocortisone | 80 mg | 80 mg |
| Prednisone | 20 mg | 100 mg |
| Prednisolone | 20 mg | 100 mg |
| Methylprednisolone | 16 mg | no effect |
| Triamcinolone | 16 mg | no effect |
| 9α fluorocortisol | 5 mg | 0.2 mg |
| Dexamethasone | 2 mg | no effect |
| DOCA | no effect | 2 mg |

Duration of Action

Cortisone acetate:    6 hour PO and IV (1/2 life
                      60-90 min.); 3 days IM
Hydrocortisone Na succinate: 4-6 hours IV (1/2 life
                      60-90 min.)
Triamcinolone:        8-12 hours PO
Dexamethasone:        8-12 hours PO
Prednisone:           6-8 hours PO

*QOD dosage advisable after initial therapy to minimize
growth retardation.

## ADRENAL MINERALOCORTICOIDS

HOW SUPPLIED:

Desoxycorticosterone acetate (DOCA):

Vials: 5 mg/ml - in oil
Pellets: 125 mg

9αFludrocortisol (Fludrocortisone):

Tablets: 0.1 mg

DOSE AND ROUTE

Desoxycorticosterone acetate:

1-3 mg/day IM (in oil) single dose
250-375 mg/year SC (implants)

9αFluorocortisol:

0.05-0.15 mg/day PO

REMARKS:

Equivalent Na Retention:

1 mg DOCA = 0.1 mg 9α-fluorocortisol.


## DOSAGES OF ANTIBIOTICS IN UREMIA

Modifications are based primarily on serum half-lives
of the antibiotics in anuric patients.

A single dose of the antibiotic is given based on a q6h,
q8h, or q12h schedule, but all subsequent doses are halved
and given at intervals based on the following table.
For example: if a child were to normally receive
10 mg/kg/day of Kanamycin as 5 mg/kg q12h, then he would
get 5 mg/kg initially but the interval before the next
dose of 2.5 mg/kg would be 36-48 hours (Clcr >10 ml/minute)
or 72-96 hours (Clcr <10 ml/minute) later.

Extreme caution must be exercised and these dosage
modifications are approximations only. Serum levels of
antibiotics at appropriate intervals should be measured
and dosage and/or interval adjusted according to serum
levels and early signs of toxicity.

ANTIBIOTICS IN UREMIA

| ANTIBIOTIC | SERUM HALF-LIFE (in Hours) | | ALSO REMOVED BY | DOSE MODIFICATION | MODIFIED DOSE INTERVAL (in Hours) in AZOTEMIA | |
|---|---|---|---|---|---|---|
| | Normal | Oliguria | | | Clcr <10 | Clcr >10 |
| Cephalothin | 0.5-0.8 | 3-18 | Liver | Minor | 24 | 12 |
| Chloramphenicol | 1.6-3.3 | 3-4 | Liver | None | - | - |
| Chlortetracycline | 5.6 | 7-11 | Liver | Do Not Use | - | - |
| Colistin | 2 | 48-72 | ? | Major | 72-96 | 36-48 |
| Erthromycin | 1.4 | 5-6 | Liver | None | - | - |
| Gentamicin | 3 | 6-20 | ? | Major | 40-56 | 12-36 |
| Kanamycin | 3 | 72-96 | ? | Major | 72-96 | 36-48 |
| Methicillin | 0.5 | 4 | Liver | None | - | - |
| Oxacillin | 0.5 | 2 | Liver | None | - | - |
| Penicillin G | 0.5 | 7-10 | Liver | Minor | 8-10 | 4-5 |
| Polymyxin B | 6 | 48-72 | ? | Major | 72-96 | 36-48 |
| Streptomycin | 2.5 | 52-100 | ? | Major | 72-96 | 36-48 |
| Tetracycline | 8.5 | 57-108 | Liver | Major | 72-96 | 36-48 |

Modified from Kunin, C.M., Annals Internal Medicine 67:151, 1967, and individual package inserts.

GUIDE FOR PREOPERATIVE MEDICATION

Before General Anesthesia

| AGE IN MONTHS | DRUGS USED |
|---|---|
| 0-6 | Atropine only |
| 6-12 | Atropine and Pentobarbital |
| over 12 | Atropine (or scopolamine) Pentobarbital Morphine (or meperidine) |

DOSAGES

Atropine (or scopolamine):
    0.02 mg/kg        - min. dose 0.15 mg
                      - max. dose 0.60 mg

Pentobarbital:
    3.0-4.0 mg/kg    - max. dose 120 mg

Morphine:
    0.05-0.10 mg/kg  - max. dose 10 mg

Meperidine:
    1.0-2.0 mg/kg    - max. dose 100 mg

Modified from J. J. Downes, Ped. Clin. N.A. 16:601, 1969.

neurologic procedures

| Age | nembutal (mg/kg) | Thorazine (mg/kg) | Demecol (mg/kg) | Atropine (mg) |
|---|---|---|---|---|
| 0-4 | 8-10 | 1.5 | 1.5 | .1 - .2 |
| 5-8 | 5-6 | 1 | 1.5 | .3 |
| 9-12+ | 2-4 | .75 | 1 | .4 |

DRUGS AND CHEMICALS TO BE AVOIDED BY PERSONS
WITH "REACTING" (PRIMAQUINE SENSITIVE) RED CELLS

Antimalarials

    1. Primaquine
    2. Pamaquine
    3. Pentaquine
    4. Plasmoquine

Sulfonamides

    1. Sulfanilamide
    2. Sulfapyridine
    3. Sulfisoxazole (Gantrisin)
    4. Salicylazosulfapyridine (Azulfidine)
    5. Sulfamethoxypryridazine (Kynex, Midicel)
    6. Sulfacetamide (Sulamyd)
    7. Trisulfapyrimidine

Nitrofurans

    1. Nitrofurantoin (Furadantin)
    2. Furazolidone (Furoxone)
    3. Furaltadone (Altafur)

Antipyretics and Analgesics

    1. Acetylsalicylic Acid
    2. Acetanilide
    3. Acetophenetidin (Phenacetin)
    4. Antipyrine
    5. Aminopyrine (Pyramidon)
    6. p-Aminosalicylic Acid

Others

    1. Sulfoxone
    2. Naphthalene
    3. Methylene Blue
    4. Phenylhydrazine
    5. Acetylphenylhydrazine
    6. Probenecid
    7. Fava Bean

NOTE: Many other compounds have been tested, but are free of hemolytic activity. Penicillin, chloromycetin, the tetracyclines, and erythromycin, for example, will not cause hemolysis. Also, the incidence of allergic reactions in these individuals is not any greater than that observed in normals. Any drug, therefore, which is not included in the list known to cause hemolysis, may be given.

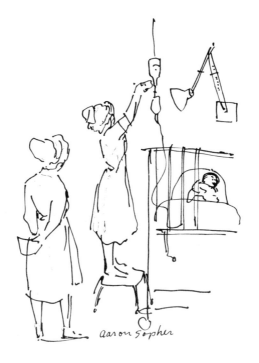

F L U I D   A N D
E L E C T R O L Y T E   T H E R A P Y

## A.  GENERAL CONSIDERATIONS

### 1.  Atomic Weights

| | | | |
|---|---|---|---|
| Aluminum (Al) | 26.97 | Magnesium (Mg) | 24.32 |
| Antimony (Sb) | 121.76 | Manganese (Mn) | 54.93 |
| Arsenic (As) | 74.91 | Mercury (Hg) | 200.61 |
| Barium (Ba) | 137.36 | Nickel (Ni) | 58.69 |
| Bismuth (Bi) | 209.00 | Nitrogen (N) | 14.01 |
| Bromine (Br) | 79.92 | Oxygen (O) | 16.00 |
| Cadmium (Cd) | 112.41 | Phosphorus (P) | 30.98 |
| Calcium (Ca) | 40.08 | Porcelain | 999.01 |
| Carbon (C) | 12.01 | Potassium (K) | 39.10 |
| Chlorine (Cl) | 35.46 | Radium (Ra) | 226.05 |
| Cobalt (Co) | 58.94 | Radon (Rn) | 222.00 |
| Copper (Cu) | 63.57 | Silicon (Si) | 28.06 |
| Fluorine (F) | 19.00 | Silver (Ag) | 107.88 |
| Gold (Au) | 197.20 | Sodium (Na) | 23.00 |
| Helium (He) | 4.00 | Sulfur (S) | 32.06 |
| Hydrogen (H) | 1.01 | Thorium (Th) | 232.12 |
| Iodine (I) | 126.92 | Tin (Sn) | 118.70 |
| Iron (Fe) | 55.85 | Uranium (U) | 238.07 |
| Lead (Pb) | 207.21 | Zinc (Zn) | 65.38 |

### 2.  Ion Calculations

a.  Moles:

Mole       = molecular weight in grams
Millimole  = molecular weight in milligrams

```
    Na 23
    Cl 35.5
    NaCl 58.5 gm = 1 mole
         58.5 mg = 1 mM
```

b.  Equivalents:

Equivalent = atomic weight divided by
                valence
mEq        = equivalent weight in mg
$\mu$Eq        = equivalent weight in $\mu$g

$Na+$ = 23/1
    23 gm Na = 1 Eq
    23 mg Na = 1 mEq

For single valence ions 1 mM = mEq.
For divalent ions 1 mM = 2 mEq.

c. Osmolality:

Osmol = atomic weight divided by number of particles exerting osmotic pressure

| | | |
|---|---|---|
| 1 mM Na+ | = 1 mOsm | |
| 1 mM NaCl | = 2 mOsm | (Na+ + Cl-) |
| 1 mM $Na_2SO_4$ | = 3 mOsm | (2Na+ + $SO_4$=) |

Osmolality is the preferred term rather than osmolarity and represents solute concentration per unit solvent (water) rather than solution (serum).

3. Conversion Factors

The following table gives factors for conversion of concentrations expressed in milliequivalents per liter to milligrams per 100 milliliters, and vice versa, for common ions that occur in physiologic solutions.

| Element or Radical | mEq per Liter | Mg per 100 ml | Mg per 100 ml | mEq per Liter |
|---|---|---|---|---|
| Sodium | 1 | 2.30 | 1 | 0.4348 |
| Potassium | 1 | 3.91 | 1 | 0.2558 |
| Calcium | 1 | 2.01 | 1 | 0.4988 |
| Magnesium | 1 | 1.22 | 1 | 0.8230 |
| Chloride | 1 | 3.55 | 1 | 0.2817 |
| Bicarbonate ($HCO_3$) | 1 | 6.10 | 1 | 0.1639 |
| Phosphorus (valence 1) | 1 | 3.10 | 1 | 0.3226 |
| Phosphorus (valence 1.8) | 1 | 1.72 | 1 | 0.5814 |
| Sulfur (valence 2) | 1 | 1.60 | 1 | 0.6250 |

Example: To convert milliequivalents of magnesium per liter to milligrams per 100 milliliters, multiply by the factor 1.22.

To convert milligrams of potassium per 100 milliliters to milliequivalents per liter, multiply by the factor 0.2558.

B. CALCULATION OF MAINTENANCE REQUIREMENTS

1. Principle

Water and electrolyte requirements are based on caloric expenditure.

2. Calculation of Caloric Expenditure for Maintenance Therapy

   a. Standard Basal Calories:

STANDARD BASAL CALORIES

| Weight Kg | Calories/24 Hours | Male and Female |
|---|---|---|
| 3 | 140 | |
| 5 | 270 | |
| 7 | 400 | |
| 9 | 500 | |
| 11 | 600 | |
| 13 | 650 | |
| 15 | 710 | |
| 17 | 780 | |
| 19 | 830 | |
| 21 | 880 | |
| 25 | 1020 | 960 |
| 29 | 1120 | 1040 |
| 33 | 1210 | 1120 |
| 37 | 1300 | 1190 |
| 41 | 1350 | 1260 |
| 45 | 1410 | 1320 |
| 49 | 1470 | 1380 |
| 53 | 1530 | 1440 |
| 57 | 1590 | 1500 |
| 61 | 1640 | 1560 |

   b. Increment for Temperature:

   Add 12% of above for each degree centigrade (8% for each degree Fahrenheit) above rectal temperature of 37.8°C (100°F).

   c. Increment for Activity:

   Add 0-30% of above for bed activity; e.g., coma or thrashing about.

3. Average Water and Electrolyte Expenditures Per 100 Calories Metabolized Per 24 Hours

| | USUAL | | | RANGE | | |
|---|---|---|---|---|---|---|
| ROUTE | $H_2O$ | Na | K | $H_2O$ | Na | K |
| Lungs | 15 | 0 | 0 | 10-60 | 0 | 0 |
| Skin | 40 | 0.1 | 0.2 | 20-100 | 0.1-3.0 | 0.2-1.5 |
| Stool | 5 | 0.1 | 0.2 | 0-50 | 0.1-4.0 | 0.2-3.0 |
| Urine | 65 | 3.0 | 2.0 | 0-400 | 0.2-30 | 0.4-30 |
| TOTAL | 125 | 3.2 | 2.4 | 30-610 | 0.4-37 | 0.8-34.5 |

a. In spite of 125 ml $H_2O$ being lost for every 100 cal/24 hr, the usual $H_2O$ requirement is 5-15 ml less (i.e., 110-120 ml) because of the production of endogenous $H_2O$ through oxidation of CHO, fat and protein.

b. Abnormally high values in above tables may be considered to represent abnormal losses.

4. Average Water and Electrolyte Requirements for Different Clinical States per 100 Calories Per 24 Hours

Based on data in preceding table:

| | ml $H_2O$ | mEq Na | mEq K |
|---|---|---|---|
| *Average patient receiving parenteral fluids | 110-120 | 2-4 | 2-3 |
| Anuria | 45 | 0 | 0 |
| Acute CNS infections and inflammation | 80-90 | 2-4 | 2-3 |
| Chronic renal disease with fixed specific gravity | 140 | variable | variable |
| Diabetes insipidus | Up to 400 | variable | variable |
| Hyperventilation | 120-210 | 2-4 | 2-3 |
| Heat Stress | 120-240 | variable | variable |
| High humidity environment | 80-100 | 2-4 | 2-3 |
| Paraoperative and post-operative patient | 85 | 1-2 | 0 |

*Adequate maintenance solution
Na and Cl: 30 mEq/L
K: 20 mEq/L

This is provided by:

5 or 10% invert sugar or glucose in $H_2O$.........800 ml
Isotonic saline................................200 ml
Potassium acetate concentrate (Cutter)............5 ml

OR

Dextrose 5% in 0.2% NaCl + 20 mEq/L K acetate.

C. DEFICIT THERAPY

1. Principles

a. Initial step: Rapidly expand the extra-cellular volume in order to improve the circulation and renal function. Blood is used only for shock not responding to

Ringer's lactate.
1) Ringer's lactate 20 cc/kg/1st hour.
2) Blood or plasma 10 cc/kg, if indicated.
b. Replace intracellular deficits slowly over
8-12 hours.  See table below for approximate
magnitude or deficits.
c. Maintenance therapy for usual losses.
d. Replace continued abnormal losses.

2.  Calculation of Deficits

PROBABLE DEFICITS OF WATER AND ELECTROLYTES IN
INFANTS WITH SEVERE DEHYDRATION (10-12 PER CENT)

| Condition | $H_2O$ ml | Na mEq | K* mEq | Cl mEq |
|---|---|---|---|---|
| | Per Kg of Body Weight | | | |
| Fasting and thirsting | 100-120 | 5-7 | 1-2 | 4-6 |
| Diarrhea | | | | |
|   Isotonic | 100-120 | 8-10 | 8-10 | 8-10 |
|   Hypertonic | 100-120 | 2-4 | 0-4 | -2 - 6** |
|   Hypotonic | 100-120 | 10-12 | 8-10 | 10-12 |
| Pyloric stenosis | 100-120 | 8-10 | 10-12 | 10-12 |
| Diabetic acidosis | 100-120 | 8-10 | 5-7 | 6-8 |

*Converted for breakdown of tissue cells:
 -1 gm N = 3 mEq of K.
**Negative balance of chloride indicates excess at
 beginning of therapy.

3.  Correction of Persistent Symptomatic
Disturbances of Electrolyte Concentration

Formula:  (CD - CA) x fD x Wt in Kg = mEq required

CD = concentration desired (mEq/L)
CA = concentration present (mEq/L)
fD = apparent distribution factor as fraction
of body weight

| Electrolyte | Apparent Distribution Factor (fD) |
|---|---|
| Bicarbonate | 0.4-0.5 |
| Chloride | 0.2-0.3 |
| Sodium | 0.6-0.7 |

D. REPLACEMENT OF CONCURRENT LOSSES IN ADDITION TO MAINTENANCE REQUIREMENTS

COMPOSITION OF EXTERNAL ABNORMAL LOSSES*

| Fluid | Na | K | Cl | Protein |
|---|---|---|---|---|
| | | mEq/L | | Gm% |
| Gastric | 20-80 | 5-20 | 100-150 | ---- |
| Pancreatic | 120-140 | 5-15 | 90-120 | ---- |
| Small intestine | 100-140 | 5-15 | 90-130 | ---- |
| Bile | 120-140 | 5-15 | 80-120 | ---- |
| Ileostomy | 45-135 | 3-15 | 20-115 | ---- |
| Diarrheal | 10-90 | 10-80 | 10-110 | ---- |
| Sweat | | | | |
| Normal | 10-30 | 3-10 | 10-35 | ---- |
| Cystic fibrosis | 50-130 | 5-25 | 50-110 | ---- |
| Burns | 140 | 5 | 110 | 3-5 |

*These losses should be determined q6h-q8h.

E. MISCELLANEOUS APPROXIMATIONS FOR BODY FLUIDS

1. Blood volume in ml = 0.08 x body weight in grams
   (0.10 x body weight for newborns and infants)

2. Quantity of packed RBC needed to raise hematocrit

$$\frac{(\text{Blood volume x desired HCT})-(\text{B.V.-present HCT})}{\text{HCT of packed RBC's}}$$

   NOTE: Most packed RBC's have a HCT in the range of 60-70%.

3. Average Platelet Increase with Platelet Transfusion

   1 unit of platelets will increase the platelet count $12 \times 10^3/m^2$ or 200/kg.

4. Average Initial Increase in Factor VIII and Factor IX Transfusions.
   2% increase/unit/kg.

5. Approximate Serum Osmolality
$$2 \text{ (Na+)} + \frac{\text{Glucose mg\%}}{18} + \frac{\text{BUN mg\%}}{2.8}$$

COMPOSITION OF FREQUENTLY USED ORAL SOLUTIONS

| Liquid | CHO | Prot.* | Calories per L. | Na | K | Cl | HCO3** | Ca | P‡ |
|---|---|---|---|---|---|---|---|---|---|
| | gm/100 ml | | | | | x mEq/l | | | |
| Milk (whole)................ | 4.9 | 3.5 | 670 | 22 | 36 | 28 | 30 | 60 | 54 |
| Milk (skim)................. | 5.5 | 3.5 | 375 | 23 | 43 | 29 | - | 61.8 | 56.9 |
| Coca cola................... | 10.9 | | 435 | 0.4 | 13 | | 13.4 | - | - |
| Pepsi-Cola.................. | 12.0 | | 480 | 6.5 | 0.8 | | 7.3 | - | - |
| 7-Up....................... | 10.15 | | 411 | 7.0 | 0.5 | | 0 | 5 | - |
| Ginger ale................. | 9.0 | | 360 | 3.5 | 0.1 | | 3.6 | 2.7 | - |
| Orange juice (sweetened).... | 14.0 | | 540 | 0.2 | 49 | | 50 | - | - |
| Grape juice................ | 18.0 | | 670 | 0.4 | 31 | | 32 | - | - |
| Tomato juice (canned and salted)... | 4.3 | | 210 | 100 | 59 | 150 | 10 | 3 | 9 |
| Apple juice................ | 14.3 | | 522 | 1.9 | 26.6 | | - | - | - |
| Lytren..................... | 7.0 | | 280 | 25 | 25 | 30 | 18 | 4 | 5 |
| HLH mixture................ | 5.0 | | 200 | 30 | 20 | 30 | 20 | 0 | 0 |
| Pedialyte.................. | 5.0 | | 200 | 30 | 20 | 30 | 14 | 4 | 0 |
| H2O (Baltimore City)....... | - | | - | 3 | 0.5 | 4 | - | - | - |

* Protein or amino acid equivalent
** Actual or potential bicarbonate, such as lactate, citrate, or acetate
‡ Calculated according to valence of 1.8
x Approximate values: actual values may vary somewhat in various localities depending on electrolyte composition of water supply used to reconstitute solution.

## COMPOSITION OF FREQUENTLY USED PARENTERAL FLUIDS

| Liquid | CHO gm/100 ml | Prot.* gm/100 ml | Calories per L. | Na (x mEq/L) | K (x mEq/L) | Cl (x mEq/L) | HCO3** (x mEq/L) | Ca (x mEq/L) | P‡ (x mEq/L) |
|---|---|---|---|---|---|---|---|---|---|
| D5W............ | 5 | – | 200 | – | – | – | – | – | – |
| D10W........... | 10 | – | 400 | – | – | – | – | – | – |
| Isotonic (normal) saline.. | – | – | – | 154 | – | 154 | – | – | – |
| 1/2 isotonic saline...... | – | – | – | 77 | – | 77 | – | – | – |
| D5 1/5 isotonic saline.... | 5 | – | 200 | 31 | – | 31 | – | – | – |
| 5% saline............ | – | – | – | 850 | – | 850 | – | – | – |
| M/6 sodium lactate....... | – | – | – | 167 | – | 167 | – | – | – |
| 3.75% sodium bicarbonate... | – | – | – | 446 | – | 446 | – | – | – |
| Ringer's............. | 0-10 | – | 0-400 | 147 | 4 | 155.5 | – | 4.5 | – |
| Ringer's lactate........ | 0-10 | – | 0-44 | 130 | 4 | 109 | 28 | 3 | – |
| Darrow's KNL.......... | – | – | – | 122 | 35 | 104 | 53 | – | – |
| Amigen 5%............ | 5-10 | 5 | 345-515 | 30 | 15 | 22 | – | 5 | 30 |
| Casein Hydrol 5%........ | – | 5 | 200 | 39 | 18 | – | – | – | – |
| Dextran 6%........... | 0-5 | 5 | 0-200 | – | – | – | – | – | – |
| Plasma (ACD).......... | – | 5 | – | 146 | 5 | 75 | 60 | – | 3 |

\* Protein or amino acid equivalent
\*\* Actual or potential bicarbonate, such as lactate, citrate, or acetate
‡ Calculated according to valence of 1.8
x Approximate values: actual values may vary somewhat in various localities depending on electrolyte composition of water supply used to reconstitute solution.

## CALCIUM SUPPLEMENTATION TO FORMULAS

| Formula | CALCIUM LACTATE (Powder = 13% Ca++) Added amt. Ca lactate (gms) per 100 cc formula: Ca/P RATIO DESIRED | | | CALCIUM GLUCONATE (1 gm/4cc) (Neocalglucon = 9% Ca++) Added amt. Neocalglucon (cc) per oz. formula: Ca/P RATIO DESIRED | | |
|---|---|---|---|---|---|---|
| | 4:1 | 3:1 | 2:1 | 4:1 | 3:1 | 2:1 |
| Similac 13 | .76 | .48 | .21 | 1.30 | .83 | .35 |
| Similac 20 | .88 | .55 | .22 | 1.50 | .93 | .37 |
| Similac 24 | 1.39 | .88 | .38 | 2.37 | 1.50 | .64 |
| Similac 27 | 1.56 | 1.00 | .42 | 2.66 | 1.69 | .72 |
| Enfamil 13 | .65 | .42 | .19 | 1.10 | .71 | .32 |
| Enfamil 20 | 1.00 | .65 | .29 | 1.70 | 1.10 | .50 |
| Enfamil 24 | 1.20 | .78 | .35 | 2.05 | 1.32 | .60 |
| Premature form. 24 | 1.72 | 1.10 | .48 | 2.92 | 1.87 | .83 |
| Nutramigen | .97 | .61 | .24 | 1.65 | 1.03 | .41 |
| Isomil | 1.00 | .62 | .23 | 1.70 | 1.05 | .39 |
| Pregestimil | .97 | .61 | .24 | 1.65 | 1.03 | .41 |
| Portagen | .97 | .61 | .24 | 1.65 | 1.03 | .41 |
| Prosobee | 1.00 | .61 | .20 | 1.72 | 1.03 | .34 |
| PM 60/40 | .31 | .15 | -- | .52 | .26 | -- |
| SMA | .64 | .40 | .16 | 1.08 | .68 | .27 |
| Cow's milk | 2.00 | 1.24 | .51 | 3.35 | 2.10 | .86 |
| Breast milk | .24 | .11 | -- | .40 | .19 | -- |
| Skim milk | 2.15 | 1.38 | .60 | 3.67 | 2.35 | 1.02 |

(Calculate amount extra calcium needed in mg/L, multiply by 0.000769)

(Calculate amount extra calcium needed in mg/L, multiply by 0.00131)

# POISONING

A. SUBSTANCES ADSORBED BY ACTIVATED CHARCOAL

Activated charcoal has been shown to be an
effective complexing agent for many drugs and
household poisons. The exact dose is as yet unknown
but present data suggests that about 1 gm/kg is an
effective dose. It is given, either PO or by nasogastric tube, as a suspension of fine powder in
enough water to produce a slurry.

## Inorganic Substances

Antimony (Sb)
Arsenic (As)
Iodine (I)
Lead (Pb)
Mercuric
  chloride ($HgCl_2$)

Phosphorus (P)
Potassium
  permanganate ($KMnO_4$)
Silver (Ag)
Tin (Sn)
Titanium (Ti)

## Organic Substances

Aconite
Alcohol
Antipyrene
Amphetamine
Atropine
Barbiturates
Cantharides
Camphor
Chloroquine
Chlorpheniramine
Chlorpromazine
Cocaine
Delphinium
Diphenylhydantoin
Digitalis
Elaterin
Ergotamine
Ethchlorvynol
Glutethimide
Hemlock
Ipecac
Kerosene

Metanamic Acid
Methylene Blue
Morphine
Muscarine
Nicotine
Opium
Oxalates
Parathione
Penicillin
Phenolphthalein
Phenol
Primaquine
Probenicid
Propoxyphene
Quinidine
Quinine
Salicylates
Stramonium
Strychnine
Sulfonamides
Veratrum

Adapted from J. Ped. 63:707, 1963
            Ped. Clin. N.A. 17:537, 1970.

B. PERITONEAL DIALYSIS (see page 117)

1. Substances which can be peritoneally dialyzed:

| | |
|---|---|
| Alcohols | Bromides |
| Ammonia | Calcium |
| Amphetamines | Chloral hydrate |
| Aniline | Diphenylhydantoin |
| Arsenic | Ethchlorvynol |
| Antibiotics | Meprobamate |
| - Carbenicillin | Potassium |
| - Isoniazid | Quinidine |
| - Kanamycin | Salicylates |
| - Neomycin | Sodium |
| Barbiturates | Strychnine |

2. Substances in which peritoneal dialysis is <u>NOT</u> effective:

| | |
|---|---|
| Antidepressants | Hallucinogens |
| Chlordiazepoxide | Lead |
| Diazepam | Magnesium |
| Digitalis | Opiates |
| Diphenylhydramine | Phenothiazines |
| Glutethimide | Propoxyphene |
| | Uric acid |

C. SALICYLATE POISONING

1. <u>Tests for Salicylate</u>

a. <u>Screening Test for Serum Salicylate</u>:
Serum from a hematocrit tube is placed on
a Phenistix. A brownish color (about 25-
50 mgm%) to purple color (about 150 mgm%)
indicates the presence of salicylate in
the serum. The diagnosis and/or therapy of
salicylate poisoning should not be based
on this screening test alone.

b. <u>Presumptive Urine Test</u>: 3 ml of urine and
3 ml of 10% ferric chloride are mixed.
A burgundy red color develops. Diacetic
acid also gives a positive test. Diacetic
acid can be removed by heating urine prior
to adding the ferric chloride. A positive
reaction after heating the urine indicates
the presence of salicylates.

<u>Ref</u>: J. Ped. <u>63</u>: 949, 1963.

SALICYLATE NOMOGRAM

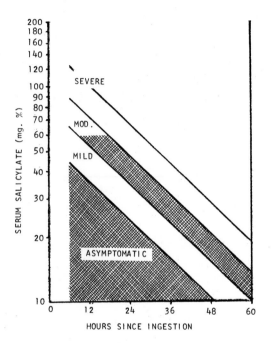

Nomogram relating serum salicylate concentration and expected severity of intoxication at varying intervals following the ingestion of a <u>single</u> dose of salicylate. (Ped. <u>26</u>:800, 1960.)

<u>NOTE</u>: In chronic salicylate overdose, overt toxicity may be manifest at much lower serum salicylate levels.

2. <u>Treatment</u>

Empty patient's stomach by means of ipecac or
lavage. Instill activated charcoal.

a. <u>Early Therapy:</u>
   1) Rapidly expand intravascular volume
      if signs of shock are present.
   2) Fluid: 160-180 ml/100 calories
      (5-10% carbohydrate) <u>plus maintenance
      and replacement of estimated deficit
      and ongoing losses</u>.
   3) Electrolytes: Na 6-8 mEq/100 calories
                    K 4-6 mEq/100 calories
   4) Alkalinization of Urine: Bicarbonate
      2 mEq/kg given over one hour. Urine
      kept alkaline with additional sodium
      and potassium bicarbonate 2 mEq/kg of
      each over next 8 hours.

   <u>NOTE:</u> Follow arterial blood gasses and
         urine pH. Give more bicarbonate to
         maintain urine pH of 7.5.

   <u>NOTE:</u> Na given as bicarbonate should be
         calculated as part of 6-8 mEq/100
         calories of Na given above.

   5) Vitamin K: IM (See Formulary for dose)

b. <u>Method of Finberg - Using Acetazolamide:</u>
   1) IV M/6 Na lactate or NaHCO3 in D5W at
      20 ml/kg/hr until urine pH is 7.5.
   2) Acetazolamide 5 mg/kg subcutaneously
      immediately after IV started.
   3) After diuresis established, change IV
      solution to contain:
          Na 40-50 mEq/liter
          K 20 mEq/liter
          50% of anion as Cl and
          50% as bicarbonate or lactate
      Adjust rate to provide water at about
      2-3 times the ordinary maintenance
      allowance.
   4) Repeat Acetazolamide 5 mg/kg for two
      additional doses at six hour intervals.
   5) Follow arterial blood gasses and
      urinary pH.

   <u>NOTE:</u> Acetazolamide may aggravate existing
         systemic acidemia or hypokalemia.

   <u>Ref:</u> Adapted from Current Pediatric
        Therapy <u>6</u>:743, 1973.

D. POTASSIUM INTOXICATION

    1. Treatment

        a. If <u>serious</u> electrocardiographic abnormali-
ties exist (pg. 70) give 10% Ca gluconate
1-2 ml/kg IV slowly with constant monitoring.

        b. Sodium bicarbonate 2 mEq/kg in 1 hour
as M/2 NaHCO₃.

        c. Exchange resin enema (see Kayexalate -
Drug Doses).

        d. <u>IF NEEDED</u>: Insulin 0.2 units/kg with
glucose 200-400 mg/kg.

E. IRON INTOXICATION

    1. Diagnosis

        a. <u>Desferal Challenge Test</u>:
Give Desferal 1 gram <u>IM</u>. Significant iron
ingestion is usually associated with a "Vin
Rose" color of the urine due to excretion
of the Desferal - iron complex.

        This test should not be used if the patient
is already in coma or shock from presumed
iron poisoning.

    2. Treatment

        a. Induce vomiting with ipecac and/or gastric
lavage with sodium bicarbonate depending on
state of consciousness. Instill Desferal
5-8 grams by stomach tube.

        b. <u>Parenteral Desferal</u>:
          1) Patients not in shock: Following
Desferal challenge test give 500 mg
Desferal <u>IM</u> q4 hours x 2 doses, then
500 mg <u>IM</u> q4-12 hours.
          2) Patients in shock: Do not give Desferal
challenge test. Give Desferal <u>IV</u> in
same dosage as above but the <u>rate of
infusion</u> should <u>not</u> exceed 15 mg/kg/hr.

        c. IV fluids and/or transfusions should be
given as necessary. Parenteral Desferal
is excreted almost exclusively in the urine
so it is mandatory to correct shock early.

        d. An upper GI series should be performed 6
weeks following ingestion.

        <u>Ref</u>: Adapted from Clinical Toxicology
<u>4</u>:615, 1971

F.  LEAD INTOXICATION

1.  Diagnosis

    Establish presumptive diagnosis using urinary
    coproporphyrin test (pg. 52 ), flat plate of
    abdomen, long bone x-rays and CBC.  Avoid lumbar
    puncture if possible.

    Definitive diagnosis made on the basis of
    blood lead level and free erythrocyte proto-
    porphyrin (FEP).

2.  Treatment

    a.  Asymptomatic:

    | Blood lead level | Treatment |
    |---|---|
    | 50-80 microgram % (FEP slightly elevated 2-3 times normal) | Follow closely especially during summer months. |
    | 50-80 microgram % (FEP markedly elevated 8-10 times normal) | EDTA 25 mg/kg/dose IM BID x 5 days, then D-Penicillamine 35-40 mg/kg/day PO in two divided doses |
    | 80-100 microgram % | EDTA 8 mg/kg/dose BAL 3 mg/kg/dose, each given IM q4h x 3 days, followed by EDTA 25 mg/kg/dose IM BID x 3 more days. Then D-Penicillamine as above. |

    Prior to chelation therapy correct dehydra-
    tion and/or electrolyte disturbances and
    establish good urine output.

    b.  Symptomatic OR blood lead level >100 micro-
        gram %

        1)  Avoid lumbar puncture if possible.
        2)  Establish urine flow cautiously
        3)  Give maintenance IV fluids at 80-90 cc/
            100 calories/24 hours (acute CNS infla-
            mation)
        4)  Control seizures

5) Then: BAL 4 mg/kg IM x 1 dose followed in 4 hours by BAL 4 mg/kg/dose and EDTA 12.5 mg/kg/dose each given IM q4h x 5-7 days. Then D-Penicillamine as above.

6) If blood lead level >80 microgram % after the first course of chelation therapy, give second course of BAL and EDTA x 5 days prior to instituting D-Penicillamine.

NOTE: Continue D-Penicillamine at above dosage until blood lead level <30 micrograms % or FEP <4 times normal.

NOTE: D-Penicillamine is contraindicated in patients with history of penicillin hypersensitivity.

Ref: Adapted from Modern Treatment 8:593, 1971

G. DIGITALIS INTOXICATION

1. Treatment
   a. Discontinue drug.
   b. Mild cases, KCl given by mouth in dose of 2-10 gm will suffice.
   c. Usual severe case: KCl by IV, given at rate of 1/2 mEq KCl/kg/hour with caution. The patient should be monitored by EKG.
   d. Stop KCl when signs of toxicity disappear or peaking of T waves becomes evident.
   e. With serious ventricular arrythmias, or where a significant overdose has been given, use Dilantin or Xylocaine (see DRUG DOSES).

BURNS

A. MANAGEMENT OF THERMAL BURNS

1. <u>Initial Procedure</u>: Perform a complete physical examination expeditiously and weigh the patient. Estimate the percentage of total body burn and record it on the burn chart. The "Rule of Nines" is not accurate for infants under 2 years of age and should be modified as shown on page 219. Consider 2nd and 3rd degree burns equally.

2. <u>Amount and Composition of Intravenous Fluids</u>

   a. <u>First 24 hour replacement</u>:
      Water - 4 ml/kg/% burn
      Na     - 0.5-0.7 mEq/kg/% burn
      These requirements are best met with Ringer's lactate. Calculate from time of burning. Half of calculated replacement volume given in first 8 hours; half in the next 16 hours.

      Colloid is not indicated in the first 24 hours.

   b. <u>Second 24 hour replacement</u>:
      One half or less of the above requirements are given in the second 24 hours. Adjust volume according to presence or absence of edema and parameters listed below.

   c. <u>Maintenance therapy</u>: A standard maintenance fluid and electrolyte regimen should be employed.

   d. <u>Relacement of nasogastric fluid loss</u>:
      Use normal saline or half normal saline. Potassium may be required.

3. <u>Patient Monitoring</u>

   Serial monitoring is the key to proper replacement and maintenance therapy. Pulse rate, central venous pressure, hematocrit, total serum solids, serum electrolytes and urinary output are necessary guidelines. With extensive burns, bladder catheterization may be necessary.

4. General Comments

   a. Give tetanus toxoid

   b. Systemic antibiotics should be used at the
      discretion of the physician. Obtain
      cultures on admission.

   c. Topical therapy is necessary to prevent
      burn wound sepsis. Topical agents in
      current use include Bentadine Ointment,
      Sulfamylon and Silver Sulfadiazine.

   d. Physical therapy to maintain range of
      motion and prevent contractures should be
      instituted in the early stages of burn
      care. Hand burns are best treated closed
      with the hand in position of function.

   Ref: Adapted from NEJM 288:444, 1973.

# BURNS

Estimate per cent of body surface involved using the
following "Rule of Nines."

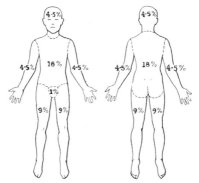

The Rule of Nines

These may have to be modified according to the patient's
age in the following manner.

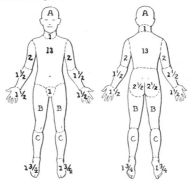

Relative percentage of areas affected by growth (After
Lund and Browder.)

| Age in years: | 0 | 1 | 5 | 10 | 15 | Adult |
|---|---|---|---|---|---|---|
| A=1/2 of head | 9-1/2 | 8-1/2 | 6-1/2 | 5-1/2 | 4-1/2 | 3-1/2 |
| B=1/2 of thigh | 2-3/4 | 3-1/4 | 4 | 4-1/4 | 4-1/2 | 4-3/4 |
| C=1/2 of 1 leg | 2-1/2 | 2-1/2 | 2-3/4 | 3 | 3-1/4 | 3-1/2 |

B.  CAUSTIC BURNS

Any pediatric patient with a history of lye ingestion should be admitted to the hospital.  Burns of
the oral pharynx and esophagus can present a serious
problem that requires the cooperation and management of several services.  In order to expedite
their disposition and care, the following procedure
is suggested:

1.  For Acute Burns (48 hours) in Children
    a.  Identify the agent.
    b.  Make the child NPO.
    c.  Start an IV.
    d.  Type and cross match severely burned
        children.
    e.  Obtain CBC, urinalysis and chest film.
    f.  Notify ENT and Pediatric Surgery services.
    g.  Perform ESOPHAGOSCOPY within 12 hours of
        burn.
    h.  Perform esophageal cinefluoroscopy within
        48 hours if possible.

2.  If No Esophageal Burn:
    a.  Child should be observed in the hospital
        for 24-48 hours.
    b.  Care for the mouth burn.
    c.  Upon discharge, the patient should be
        followed by the Pediatric Service.

3.  If Esophagus is Burned:
    a.  Steroid therapy (must be within 48 hours).
        Dose: 2 mg/kg/day of prednisone or its
        equivalent.
    b.  Antibiotics:  Ampicillin x 10 days.
        IV fluids until patient can handle secre-
        tions which is usually within 48 hours.
        Thereafter, a clear liquid diet and advance
        to soft diet as tolerated.
    d.  Further management, at this point, can
        be determined in consultation with the ENT
        and Pediatric Surgical Services.

R E S P I R A T O R Y   C A R E   A N D
P U L M O N A R Y   F U N C T I O N

GUIDE TO RESPIRATORY CARE

1. The patient should be turned side to side and side to back at least q2h. If the patient is mechanically ventilated, disconnect from ventilator for turning, then reconnect.

2. Suction should be performed PRN or at least q1h.

3. Saline instillation is best accomplished via a sterile suction catheter by injecting past the tip of the intratracheal airway as the operator brings the catheter up.

   Normal sterile saline without a bacteriostatic additive is used for intratracheal instillation. Approximate amounts used:

   | | |
   |---|---|
   | Premature - Newborn | 0.5cc |
   | Up to 1 year | 1.0cc |
   | 1 - 3 years | 2.0cc |
   | 3 - 5 years | 2.5cc |
   | 5 - 10 years | 3.0cc |
   | 10 years and older | 3.5 to 4.0cc |

4. Hyperventilation with an "ambubag" connected to a source of $O_2$ is indispensable before and after saline instillations and suctioning. Breath sounds are to be checked bilaterally before and after suction.

5. Chest physiotherapy should be performed about every four to six hours. This should include:

   Percussion to all lobes or to specifically involved lobe(s). This is usually followed by:
   Vibration, although difficult to accomplish with the hands, can be done with mechanical vibrators if available.
   Thoracic "squeezing" is performed in combination with vibration. The goal is to maximally decrease the residual volume after a deep breath (usually a manual inflation with an "ambubag" produces an excellent deep breath). By compressing the sides of the thorax, a forceful expiration is obtained. Secretions may be expressed into

222

larger airways, then suctioned.

6. Tracheal aspirates should be sent for culture q.o.d.

7. The inspired $O_2$ concentration ($FIO_2$) should be checked at least q2h.

8. Ventilator settings should be stated in the Dr.'s orders. The desired $O_2$ concentration should be determined according to the blood gases. Any change in settings should be followed by blood gas analysis.

ESTIMATION OF NASOTRACHEAL TUBE LENGTH

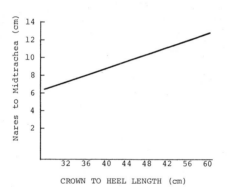

CROWN TO HEEL LENGTH (cm)

<u>Ref</u>:   Peds: 41:823, 1967.

ESTIMATION OF ENDOTRACHEAL TUBE SIZE

| Approximate Age | French Equivalent | Metric Inside Diameter |
|---|---|---|
| Premie and Small Newborn | 11-12 Fr. | 2.5 mm |
| Large Newborn up to 3 months | 13<br>15 | 3.0<br>3.5 |
| Up to 18 months | 17<br>19 | 4.0<br>4.5 |
| 18 months to 3 years | 20-21<br>22-23 | 5.0<br>5.5 |
| 3 to 5 years | 24-26 | 6.0 |
| 5 to 7 years | 26-27 | 6.5 |
| 8 to 10 years | 29-30 | 7.0 |
| 11 to 12 years | 32-33 | 7.5 |
| 12 years and older | 34-35 | 9.0 |

BLOOD MEASUREMENTS IN
VARIOUS ACID-BASE DISTURBANCES*

| | pH | PaCO2 | HCO3- (mEq/L) | CO2 Content (mEq/L) |
|---|---|---|---|---|
| NORMAL VALUES | 7.35-7.45 | 35-45 | 24-26 | 25-28 |
| Metabolic Acidosis | ↓ | ↓ | ↓ | ↓ |
| Acute Respiratory Acidosis | ↓ | ↑ | ↔ | Slight ↑ |
| Compensated Respiratory Acidosis | ↔ or slight ↓ | ↑ | ↑ | ↑ |
| Metabolic Alkalosis | ↑ | Slight ↑ | ↑ | ↑ |
| Acute Respiratory Alkalosis | ↑ | ↓ | ↔ | Slight ↓ |
| Compensated Respiratory Alkalosis | ↔ or slight ↑ | ↓ | ↓ | ↓ |

*Values obtained by arteriolized capillary blood or direct arterial puncture.

SHUNT AT DIFFERENT INSPIRED OXYGEN MIXTURES

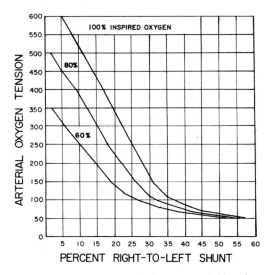

Calculations are based on an assumed hemoglobin of 16 gm%, an arteriovenous difference of 4 volumes per cent, a respiratory quotient of 0.8 and an arterial $PCO_2$ of 40 mmHg.

## PREDICTED BASAL TIDAL VOLUME

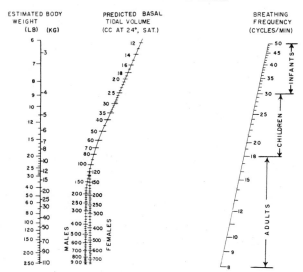

CORRECTIONS TO BE APPLIED TO PREDICTED
BASAL TIDAL VOLUME

a) When measurements are based on English system
   (lb; °F.):
   Daily activity (i.e. patients not in coma):
   add 10%
   Fever: add 5% for each °F. above 99°F. (rectal)
   Altitude: add 5% for each 2,000 feet above sea
   level.
   Tracheotomy (or endotracheal tube): subtract a
   volume equal to one-half body weight in lbs.

b) When measurements are based on Metric system:
   Daily activity: add 10%
   Fever: add 9% for each 1°C. above 37°C. (rectal)
   Altitude: add 8% for each 1,000 M above sea
   level.
   Tracheotomy (or endotracheal tube): subtract a
   volume equal to body weight (kg.)

BRONCHOPULMONARY SEGMENTS

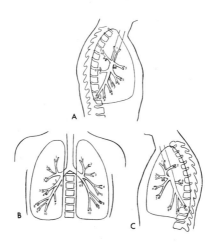

The nomenclature of bronchopulmonary anatomy, adapted from report by the Thoracic Society in 1950. (Adapted from Negus.)

| RIGHT LUNG | LEFT LUNG |
|---|---|

**RIGHT LUNG**

Upper lobe
1. Apical
2. Posterior
3. Anterior

Middle lobe
4. Lateral
5. Medial

Lower lobe
6. Apical
7. Cardiac (medial basal)
8. Anterior
9. Lateral
10. Posterior

**LEFT LUNG**

Upper lobe
1. ⎫
2. ⎬ Apicoposterior
3. Anterior

4. ⎫
5. ⎬ Lingula

Lower lobe
6. Apical
7. Absent
8. Anterior
9. Lateral ⎫
10. Posterior ⎬ Basal

228

LUNG VOLUMES

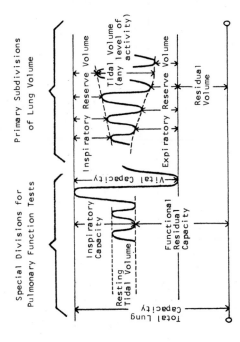

Subdivisions of Lung Volumes. Fed. Proc. 9:602, 1950

INFECTIOUS DISEASES

RECOMMENDED SCHEDULE FOR ACTIVE
IMMUNIZATION OF INFANTS AND CHILDREN
Modified from the
American Academy of Pediatrics 1974

| AGE | PREPARATION |
|---|---|
| 2 months | DPT*<br>Trivalent OPV# |
| 4 months | DPT<br>Trivalent OPV |
| 6 months | DPT<br>Trivalent OPV |
| 12 months | Tuberculin Test<br>Measles Vaccine |
| 18 months | DPT<br>Trivalent OPV |
| 2-10 years | Rubella<br>Tuberculin Test every 1-2 years |
| 3 years | DPT |
| 5 years | DT+<br>Trivalent OPV |
| 12-14 years | DT<br>Mumps<br>Tuberculin Test |
| 16 years | Tuberculin Test |

After 16 years of age tetanus toxoid booster doses
should be repeated every 10 years.

*Diphtheria-Pertussis-Tetanus Toxoid
#Oral Polio Vaccine
+Diphtheria-Tetanus Toxoid

NOTE:   Interruption or delay of a series does not
        require restarting the immunizations.

A. ACTIVE IMMUNIZATION

1. <u>Diphtheria, Pertussis, and Tetanus (DPT)</u>

Precipitated or adsorbed triple vaccine:
usual dose 0.5 ml. Start course between 6 and
8 weeks of age, giving injections 1 to 3 months
apart, although up to 6 months may lapse
between injections. Give boosters at ages 1-1/2
and 3 years, then adult type diphtheria-tetanus
vaccine until age 12, as indicated in preceding
table.

a. <u>Precautions:</u>
1) Defer in presence of any active infection.
2) In infant who has had febrile con-
vulsions, start with fractional doses,
(0.1-0.25 ml), and give aspirin.
3) If previous injection has produced high
fever, somnolence, or unusual reactions,
reduce dosage subsequently.
4) If convulsion or other severe reaction
has occurred, discontinue pertussis,
and try fractional doses of separate
diphtheria and tetanus antigens.
5) Presence of cerebral damage is an
indication for delaying active
immunization until 1 year of age.
Use fractional doses with single antigens.
b. <u>Special Situations:</u>
1) If child has had proven pertussis,
use D-T only. (Parapertussis has no
cross-immunity.)
2) Over age 3 years use DT antigen ("adult
type"). Using 0.5 ml dosage, prelimi-
nary Schick and toxoid sensitivity
tests are unnecessary.
3) To attempt rapid immunization of young
infants in the face of a pertussis
outbreak, use fluid pertussis vaccine,
0.5 ml subcutaneously once a week x 3.
This schedule does not provide as good
immunity as longer spacing or depot
vaccines.

c. Guide To Tetanus Prophylaxis in Wound Management:

| History of Tetanus Immunization (Doses) | Clean, Minor Wounds | | All Other Wounds | |
|---|---|---|---|---|
| | Toxoid | Tetanus Immune Globulin | Toxoid | Tetanus Immune Globulin |
| Uncertain | Yes | No | Yes | Yes |
| 0-1 | Yes | No | Yes | Yes |
| 2 | Yes | No | Yes | No[1] |
| 3 or more | No[2] | No | No[3] | No |

1. Unless wound more than 24 hours old.
2. Unless more than 10 years since last dose.
3. Unless more than 5 years since last dose.

Ref: U.S.P.H.S.: Weekly Morbidity and Mortality Report, Vol. 20, No. 43, 1971.

2. Poliomyelitis

Live Vaccine: Provided as trivalent vaccine and administered orally only. Storage and dose instructions vary with manufacturer and must be adhered to. Immunization of infants may be started as young as 6 weeks of age, but a combined dose for all three types is recommended six months later to allow multiplication of any one type which might have been suppressed by passive immunity of infancy. Trivalent boosters are currently given at 18 months and 5 years.

Contraindications:
a. Immunodeficiency disease or immuno-suppressive therapy
b. Malignancy
c. Pregnancy

3. Measles

Give live, attenuated measles virus vaccine 0.5 cc SC (Schwartz or Moraten) into deltoid.

Contraindications:
a. Leukemia and other malignancies
b. Febrile illness
c. History of egg sensitivity
d. Defer during polio epidemic
e. Pregnancy

f.  When PPD positive, vaccine may be given,
    but the patient should be placed on
    antituberculous therapy prior to
    vaccination.
g.  Defer until 8 weeks after any adminis-
    tration of blood plasma or immune
    globulin.

NOTE:  Systemic manifestations may occur
between the 5th and 12th day.

4.  Smallpox

No longer routinely recommended but suggested for people at high risk such as
travelers to and from countries where
smallpox is epidemic as well as for health
service personnel.

Ref:  U.S.P.H.S.:  Weekly Morbidity and
Mortality Report, Vol. 20, No. 38, 1971.

Use calf lymph virus, kept frozen until use,
and the multiple puncture technique, over
the insertion of the left deltoid.  The
lesion should be kept dry, and no dressing
used.  Inspect primary vaccinations at 8
to 10 days, and revaccinations at 4 to 7
days.
a.  Primary Vaccinia:  Maximal erythema in
    8 to 14 days.  Progression:  Vesicle to
    pustule to crust to scar.  Indicates
    complete absence of previous immunity.
b.  Vaccinoid Reaction:  Maximal erythema
    in 4 to 7 days.  Virus propagation occurs
    but is terminated by accelerated recall
    of immunity.  Usually a mild scar is pro-
    duced.
c.  Early Reaction:  Maximal erythema between
    8 and 72 hours.  No scar produced.  This
    reaction indicates good immunity only if
    the lot of vaccine is proven to be live
    by production of primary vaccinia in
    other patients.  If virus is dead, this
    reaction indicates sensitivity to protein
    but not necessarily immunity.
d.  No Reaction:  An indication of an unsuc-
    cessful attempt, not of immunity, and
    should be repeated.

Special Situations:
1)  Annual vaccination is necessary for
    optimal protection as in endemic areas.

2) The Surgeon General recommends vaccination of medical personnel every three years because of present rapid world-wide travel.

3) Rapid recall is best produced by revaccination on the flexor surface of the forearm. (See also passive immunization.)

Contraindications to Vaccination:
1) Dermatitis (especially eczema) in the patient or his household.
2) Steroid, x-ray, and antimetabolite therapy are contraindications as are certain neoplastic diseases and immuno-logic deficiency diseases.
3) Pregnancy.

Complications of Vaccination: The American Academy of Pediatric's Report of the Committee on Infectious Diseases, ("Redbook"), contains a list of individuals with access to vaccinia immune globulin.

5. Influenza

Bivalent A and B vaccine is available, but the antigenic makeup of the vaccine varies from year to year. Primary course is 2 injections, given subcutaneously except when the dose is less than 0.2 ml, in which case better response is obtained with intra-dermal injection. Age 3 months to 6 years: 0.1 to 0.2 ml at 1 to 2 week interval, with a booster 3 months later. Age 6 to 12 years: 0.5 ml on 2 occasions 2 or more months apart. Adults: 1.0 ml on 2 occasions 2 or more months apart. Give a booster each fall. This vaccine is contraindicated in patients with egg sensitivity.

Indications: Not routinely recommended for pediatric patients. Every year in patients with chronic debilitating cardiovascular, pulmonary, renal or metabolic disorders, especially congenital heart disease, cystic fibrosis, Addison's disease, chronic asthma, TB, diabetes. Also recommended for pregnant women. In epidemic years many other groups such as health and hospital workers may be candidates for immunization, depending on current opinion.

6. Mumps

   Inactivated: Not recommended for routine
   use in healthy children. Degree and duration
   of immunity not clearly established.

   Live Attenuated: Recommended for children
   approaching puberty, adolescents and adults
   who have not had clinical disease. Given
   SC only after excess antiseptic cleaned off
   skin.

   Contraindications:
   a. Egg sensitivity.
   b. Agammaglobulinemia.
   c. Patients with malignancies, or on anti-
      metabolites or steroids.
   d. Pregnancy.

7. Rabies

   The decision to treat for rabies must be
   based on whether the attack was provoked,
   the type of animal and whether it is
   available, the immunization status of the
   animal, and the presence of rabies in the
   state or community.

   After severe exposures to potentially rabid
   animals (particularly following bites about
   the head and neck), individuals should be
   given equine antirabies serum, plus active
   immunization with avian vaccine. Appropriate
   conjunctival and skin tests should be
   carried out with the equine serum. Serum
   dosage is obtained from the brochure supplied
   by the manufacturer with each vial. Active
   immunization should consist of 14 daily
   injections of the avian vaccine supplemented
   by two booster doses of avian vaccine 10 to
   20 days after the last of the daily doses.

   NOTE: A limited amount of human rabies
   immune globulin is available for persons
   at great risk of anaphylaxis to the equine
   serum. Cutter Laboratories, Berkeley,
   California should be contacted regarding
   it's availability.

8. Rocky Mountain Spotted Fever

   Recommended only for high risk persons. Cox
   yolk sac vaccine in 3 SC injections of
   of 0.5 ml each at 5 to 7 day intervals.

An annual stimulating dose will maintain a high level of protection.  Do not give to those sensitive to egg.

9.  Rubella

Live rubella vaccine is currently recommended by the American Academy of Pediatrics.  It should be given to boys and girls between 1 year of age and puberty.  It is contra-indicated in pregnancy.  Opinions vary as to its efficacy in establishing permanent immunity.

10.  Tuberculosis

BCG is given only when the PPD is negative. 0.1 ml is given subcutaneously, as super-ficially as possible, over the right deltoid, or by the multiple puncture technique of Rosenthal.  The PPD should be repeated 12 weeks after vaccination and periodically; if negative at 12 weeks, BCG is considered to have failed and should be repeated.

a.  Indications:
   1)  Newborns at risk of exposure at home should be vaccinated in the nursery and kept from exposure until PPD positive.
   2)  Children who have been exposed to TB but who can be isolated from expo-sure for 8 weeks prior to vaccination, who then still have a negative PPD, and who can be isolated following vaccination until PPD converts.
b.  Contraindications:  Premature infants or persons suffering from immuno-deficiency states, burns, impetigo or other infectious skin diseases.  Do not administer BCG simultaneously with smallpox, or with the administration of corticosteroids.

11.  Typhoid

Routine typhoid immunization is no longer recommended for the U.S.A.

Indications in special situations include:
a.  Epidemics within institutions or communities.
b.  Foreign travel to an epidemic or endemic area.

      c.  Continued close contact to a known
          carrier.

12.  <u>CHOLERA, YELLOW FEVER, PLAGUE AND TYPHUS</u>
are used only in foreign travel to affected
countries and in other high risk situations.

b.  PASSIVE IMMUNIZATION

1.  <u>Infectious Hepatitis</u>

Usual recommendation is 0.02 to 0.04 ml/kg
gamma globulin IM for both children and
adults.  Repeat dosage q6 weeks if exposure
continues.

2.  <u>Measles</u>

<u>Preventive dose</u>:  0.25 ml/kg gamma globulin
IM as soon after exposure as possible.
Indicated for children who (1) are under 3;
(2) are hospitalized; (3) are chronically
ill; (4) have siblings with other diseases
(especially TB, pertussis, rheumatic
fever).

<u>Modifying dose</u>:  0.05 ml/kg within 6 days of
exposure.  Indicated for all children and
adults with negative histories.  After an
interval of at least 6 weeks active immunization with live vaccine should be given
where not contraindicated.

3.  <u>Pertussis</u>

In non-vaccinated children under the age of
2, pertussis immune gamma globulin (human),
2.5 ml, is harmless (as opposed to hyper-
immune human serum), but this preparation is
of no proven value in either prophylaxis or
treatment.

4.  <u>Rubella</u>

20 ml gamma globulin for pregnant women
exposed during the first trimester is of
questionable benefit since rash can be
suppressed without preventing viremia and
teratogenesis.

5.  <u>Tetanus</u>

Allergic reactions are frequent following
the use of horse serum antitoxin in tetanus

prophylaxis; often the reactions are severe, occasionally they are fatal. Various alternatives such as rapid active immunization and antibiotic prophylaxis have become popular in order to avoid administering horse serum. Human tetanus hyper-immune gamma globulin (HTG) has been marketed recently, making it possible to dispense with horse antitoxin entirely.

More widespread active immunization with tetanus toxoid is strongly recommended, for active immunization before the injury obviates the need for antitoxin. If active immunization is begun after the injury (see page 231), and if HTG is also to be given at the same time it is best to use 0.5 ml fluid toxoid, waiting 3 hours before giving HTG into the other arm. Precipitated toxoids should be avoided in this situation.

HTG is more expensive than horse antitoxin, but not prohibitively so, and the increased expense is offset by the virtual elimination of allergic reactions. Because it is a homologous protein, it disappears from the serum more slowly than horse antitoxin; thus, smaller amounts are effective. A dose of 250 units HTG appears adequate in children and adults. This seems equivalent to at least 1500 units of horse antitoxin, and it gives protection for at least 1 month. It should be given intramuscularly only. This material does not transmit serum hepatitis. Antitoxin is only an adjunct to careful and thorough surgical treatment of tetanus-prone wounds.

Ref: New Eng. J. Med. 270:175, 1964.
New Eng. J. Med. 268:857, 1963.

6. Vaccinia and Smallpox

Vaccinia immune gamma globulin is now available through consultants to the American Red Cross.

Indications: Eczema vaccinatum, generalized vaccinia, vaccinia necrosum, ocular autoinoculation of vaccinia, and in conjunction with vaccination in all cases of known smallpox exposure. It has also been demonstrated to be effective in prophylaxis of children with eczema who must be vaccinated, and of children who are burned or developed varicella soon after vaccination. It has not been effective in the treatment of vaccinia encephalitis.

7. <u>Immunodeficiency Disorders</u>

<u>Gamma Globulin</u>: 0.7 ml/kg IM ql-4 weeks with a maximum dose of 20-30 ml. A double dose is given at the onset of therapy. <u>This is of no efficacy in cellular immuno-deficiency states</u>.

<u>Plasma Therapy</u>: 10-20 ml/kg, IV, q6-8 weeks. Continual plasmaphoresis of one donor is essential to reduce the risk of hepatitis. If there is deficient T-cell function, the plasma should be frozen and rethawed to avoid graft <u>vs</u> host disease.

8. <u>Rabies</u> (see page 234 under Active Immuni-zation.)

INCUBATION PERIODS AND ISOLATION PERIODS
FOR SOME COMMON CONTAGIOUS DISEASES

| Disease | Duration of Average Incubation Period | Isolation of Patient | Observation or Quarantine Of Susceptible Patients |
|---|---|---|---|
| Chickenpox | 12-16 days | Until pustules and most scabs gone, usually about 7 days. | 11-17 days from first exposure. |
| Diphtheria | Usually 2-4 days | Until two successive negative cultures of nose and throat are obtained, taken no less than 24 hours apart, nor before 7th day. | Observation for 7 days from last contact or until negative culture is obtained. Schick test for all contacts. |
| Rubeola | Usually about 10 days | Until 5 days after appearance of rash. | Observation 14 days from exposure. |
| Meningococcus meningitis | Irregular, 1-5 days | Duration of febrile period, or first 24 hrs. of effective antibiotic therapy. | Observation for 7 days from last exposure. |
| Mumps | 16-18 days | Duration of swelling. | Observation during third week from first exposure. |
| Poliomyelitis | 7-14 days | Duration of febrile period. | Observation for 2 weeks for any minor illness. |
| Rubella | 14-21 days | Duration of catarrh and rash. | Observation 12th-20th days. |

Incubation Periods and Isolation Periods for Some Common Contagious Diseases (continued)

| Disease | Duration of Average Incubation Period | Isolation of Patient | Observation or Quarantine of Susceptible Patients |
|---|---|---|---|
| Scarlet fever | Usually 2-4 days (1-7 days) | Until infection cured, at least 7 days. | Observation until 1 week from last exposure. |
| Smallpox | Usually about 12 days | Until all crusts and scabs are gone. | Quarantine 3 weeks. Rules modified by vaccination. |
| Pertussis | 7 days | Until 1 week after last paroxysm with vomiting. | For 2 weeks from last exposure. Quarantine for unvaccinated under 5 years; observation for others. |

ISOLATION TYPES AND TECHNIQUES

| DISEASE | RESPIRATORY | ENTERIC[4] | SPECIAL | | PROTECTIVE | |
|---|---|---|---|---|---|---|
| | Bacterial meningitis[2] Zoster-Chickenpox Tuberculosis Measles (Rubeola) Diphtheria Pertussis Measles (Rubella)[3] Staph pneumonia | Staph enteritis Shigella Salmonella Infant diarrhea[5] Aseptic meningitis Coxsackie Polio Echo Hepatitis[6] Serum Infectious | Staph wounds Puerperal sepsis[4] Pelvic infections (draining)[4] | Tetanus Gas bacillus Septic wounds Eye infections | Vaccinia Smallpox | Thermal burns[8] Hyper-susceptibility |
| Handwashing | Upon leaving room | Upon leaving room | Upon leaving room | Upon leaving room | Upon leaving room | Upon leaving room |
| Single Room | Yes | Yes | Yes | Not neces. | Yes[7] | Yes |
| Gown | No | Yes | Yes | No | Yes | Yes |
| Mask | Yes | No | Staph wounds only | No | Yes | Yes |

(Continued on next page)

242

Isolation Types and Techniques (Continued)

| | RESPIRATORY | ENTERIC4 | SPECIAL | | PROTECTIVE |
|---|---|---|---|---|---|
| | | | To handle soiled linen and dressings. | Yes | No |
| Gloves1 | No | No | | Yes | No |
| Care of Articles | To be discarded; or washed and disinfected; or wrapped for sterilization. | | | | Treat as non-isolation |

1. Use plastic disposable isolation-type.
2. Isolate until 24 hours after onset of treatment.
3. Pregnant nursing personnel should not care for these patients. Urine of congenitally infected infants is infective.
4. Bedpan precautions for all patients.
5. Infant diarrhea may be grouped.
6. Syringe and needle precautions.
7. Room should not be used for eczema patient for one year after these patients have occupied it.
8. Use sterile gowns and linen.

# K E T O G E N I C   D I E T

The ketogenic diet is a dietary regimen that may be of
value in the treatment of intractable grand mal or
minor motor seizures.  Best results are obtained in
children 2-5 years of age, but it may be tried up to
8 years or beyond and before 2 years of age.  It is
usually reserved for those uncontrolled by usual
anticonvulsant drugs.  Adequate parental supervision
and some cooperation by the patient are essential.

1.  Method of Starting Diet

   a.  An initial period of starvation to establish
       adequate ketosis is necessary.  This lasts a
       minimum of 3 days, usually 5-7 days.  Unless
       untoward reactions occur, intake is limited to
       400-800 ml water per day.  The diet is begun
       after the patient has lost 10% of body weight,
       and the urinary acetone and diacetic acid tests
       have been 4+ for several days.  A serum bicarbo-
       nate of <10 mEq/L or the presence of Kuss-Maul
       respirations are criteria to terminate the
       starvation period before 10% weight loss.
   b.  One-third of the calculated diet is offered on
       the first day, and then increased to 2/3, and
       finally to full rations on successive days,
       if the ketosis is not appreciably lessened.
   c.  Evaluation of the patient is both by clinical
       and by laboratory means.  Routine to be followed
       includes:
       1)  Pulse and respirations q4h.
       2)  Daily morning weights (ac, after voiding).
       3)  Urine specimens (ac, breakfast and supper)
           for urine specific gravity, acetone, and
           diacetic acid, daily.
       4)  Fasting blood sugar, $CO_2$, K, and uric acid
           to be studied on day of starvation and
           repeated in 3 days and on day of discharge.

       NOTE:  Appropriate measures are taken for
       symptoms of hypoglycemia or marked acidosis.

   d.  If anticonvulsant drugs are being given, they
       may be tapered.  If phenobarbital is used, it
       should be continued to the first ketogenic diet
       meal, and then eliminated gradually over the
       next 2 weeks.  If other drugs are being used
       with phenobarbital, they may be discontinued
       when the starvation is begun.  If phenobarbital
       is not employed, but other drugs are, they may
       be reduced daily and discontinued by the end
       of the starvation period.  Drugs should not be
       administered in a carbohydrate vehicle.

2.  Composition and Calculation of the 4:1 Diet

    a.  The diet consists of 4 grams of fat (keto-
        genic), 1 gram of protein and carbohydrate
        combined (antiketogenic).
    b.  Method of Calculation:
        1)  The 4 gm of fat plus 1 gm of protein
            plus CHO are considered a "dietary unit,"
            and yield 40 calories.
        2)  Daily caloric requirement is 60-75
            cal/kg/day, depending on age.
        3)  Determine number of "dietary units" required
            per day; i.e., total daily caloric require-
            ments divided by 40.
        4)  Calculate gm of fat/day (number of "dietary
            units" x 4).
        5)  Calculate gm of protein/day on basis of
            about 1 gm/kg/day.
        6)  Obtain gm of CHO/day by difference.
    c.  Example  (for a 5-year old, weighing 18 kg)
        1)  Daily requirement: 18 kg x 70 cal/kg =
            1260 cal/day.
        2)  Number of "dietary units":  1260 cal ÷
            40 cal/unit = 31.5 units.
        3)  Number of grams of fat:  31.5 units x
            4 gm fat/unit = 126 gm.
        4)  Number of grams of protein:  1.0 gm/kg
            x 18 kg = 18 gm.
        5)  Number of grams CHO:  31.5 gm (since protein
            plus CHO = 1 gm/unit) minus 18 = 13.5 gm.

3.  Method of Discontinuing Diet

    After 2 years on the 4:1 ratio, the diet is reduced
    to a 3:1 (ketogenic:antiketogenic) ratio from
    3 months to 1 year, and finally to a 2:1 ratio for
    another three months, after which time a normal diet
    is resumed.

    NOTE:  Urine should be checked daily for ketone
    bodies while on diet as abruptly breaking of
    ketosis may precipitate recurrence of seizures.

4.  Complications

    a.  Hypoglycemia
    b.  Uric acid nephropathy
    c.  Severe acidosis

PART IV

REFERENCE DATA

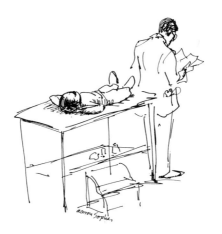

NORMAL MEASUREMENTS BY AGE

| | MALE | | | | FEMALE | | | | BOTH SEXES | |
|---|---|---|---|---|---|---|---|---|---|---|
| | HEIGHT cm. | WEIGHT kg. | UPPER LOWER SEGMENT cm. | U/L ratio | HEIGHT cm. | WEIGHT kg. | UPPER LOWER SEGMENT cm. | U/L ratio | HEAD cm. | CHEST cm. |
| BIRTH | 50.8 | 3.4 | 18.8 / 32.0 | 1.70 | 50.8 | 3.2 | 18.8 / 32.0 | 1.70 | 35.1 | 34.8 |
| 1/12 | 53.6 | 4.3 | 20.3 / 33.5 | 1.67 | 54.6 | 4.1 | 20.3 / 34.3 | 1.69 | 36.3 | 36.3 |
| 2/12 | 56.4 | 5.1 | 21.1 / 35.3 | 1.67 | 57.2 | 5.0 | 21.3 / 35.8 | 1.68 | 37.8 | 37.8 |
| 3/12 | 59.2 | 6.0 | 22.4 / 36.8 | 1.64 | 59.7 | 5.9 | 22.4 / 37.3 | 1.67 | 39.1 | 39.4 |
| 4/12 | 61.7 | 6.8 | 23.4 / 38.4 | 1.64 | 62.0 | 6.6 | 23.4 / 38.6 | 1.65 | 40.4 | 40.9 |
| 5/12 | 64.5 | 7.6 | 24.6 / 39.9 | 1.62 | 64.0 | 7.3 | 24.4 / 39.6 | 1.62 | 41.7 | 42.4 |
| 6/12 | 67.3 | 8.5 | 25.7 / 41.7 | 1.62 | 65.5 | 7.7 | 25.1 / 40.4 | 1.61 | 43.2 | 43.9 |
| 7/12 | 68.8 | 8.9 | 26.4 / 42.4 | 1.61 | 67.1 | 8.2 | 25.9 / 41.1 | 1.59 | 43.7 | 44.5 |
| 8/12 | 70.4 | 9.3 | 27.2 / 43.2 | 1.59 | 68.6 | 8.6 | 26.7 / 41.9 | 1.57 | 44.2 | 44.7 |
| 9/12 | 71.9 | 9.6 | 27.9 / 43.9 | 1.57 | 70.1 | 9.0 | 27.4 / 42.7 | 1.56 | 45.0 | 45.2 |
| 10/12 | 73.2 | 10.0 | 28.4 / 44.7 | 1.57 | 71.4 | 9.3 | 28.0 / 43.2 | 1.53 | 45.5 | 45.7 |
| 11/12 | 74.7 | 10.4 | 29.2 / 45.5 | 1.56 | 72.9 | 9.6 | 29.0 / 43.9 | 1.52 | 46.0 | 46.0 |
| 12/12 | 76.2 | 10.8 | 30.0 / 46.2 | 1.54 | 74.2 | 10.0 | 29.5 / 44.7 | 1.52 | 46.5 | 46.5 |
| 1&1/12 | 77.2 | 11.0 | 30.5 / 46.7 | 1.53 | 75.2 | 10.2 | 30.0 / 45.2 | 1.51 | 46.7 | 46.7 |
| 2/12 | 78.0 | 11.3 | 31.0 / 47.0 | 1.52 | 76.2 | 10.5 | 30.5 / 45.7 | 1.50 | 47.0 | 47.0 |
| 3/12 | 79.0 | 11.5 | 31.5 / 47.5 | 1.51 | 77.2 | 10.7 | 31.0 / 46.2 | 1.49 | 47.2 | 47.2 |
| 4/12 | 79.8 | 11.8 | 31.8 / 48.0 | 1.51 | 78.2 | 10.9 | 31.5 / 46.7 | 1.48 | 47.8 | 47.5 |
| 5/12 | 80.8 | 12.0 | 32.3 / 48.5 | 1.50 | 79.2 | 11.1 | 32.0 / 47.2 | 1.48 | 48.0 | 47.8 |
| 6/12 | 81.8 | 12.4 | 32.8 / 49.0 | 1.49 | 80.0 | 11.4 | 32.5 / 47.5 | 1.46 | 48.3 | 48.0 |
| 7/12 | 82.8 | 12.6 | 33.0 / 49.5 | 1.49 | 81.0 | 11.6 | 33.3 / 47.8 | 1.44 | 48.3 | 48.3 |
| 8/12 | 83.8 | 12.6 | 33.8 / 50.0 | 1.48 | 82.0 | 11.8 | 33.8 / 48.3 | 1.43 | 48.5 | 48.5 |
| 9/12 | 84.6 | 12.8 | 34.5 / 50.0 | 1.45 | 83.1 | 12.0 | 34.3 / 48.8 | 1.42 | 48.5 | 48.8 |

NORMAL MEASUREMENTS BY AGE (continued)

| | MALE | | | | | FEMALE | | | | | BOTH SEXES | |
|---|---|---|---|---|---|---|---|---|---|---|---|---|
| | HEIGHT | WEIGHT | UPPER | LOWER | U/L | HEIGHT | WEIGHT | UPPER | LOWER | U/L | HEAD | CHEST |
| | | | SEGMENT | | ratio | | | SEGMENT | | ratio | | |
| | cm. | kg. | cm. | | | cm. | kg. | cm. | | | cm. | cm. |
| 10/12 | 85.6 | 12.9 | 50.5 | 35.1 | 1.44 | 84.1 | 12.2 | 49.3 | 34.8 | 1.42 | 48.5 | 49.0 |
| 11/12 | 86.6 | 13.1 | 51.1 | 35.6 | 1.44 | 85.1 | 12.4 | 49.8 | 35.3 | 1.41 | 48.8 | 49.3 |
| 12/12 | 87.4 | 13.3 | 51.3 | 36.1 | 1.42 | 86.1 | 12.5 | 50.3 | 35.8 | 1.40 | 48.8 | 49.5 |
| 2&6/12 | 92.2 | 14.3 | 53.3 | 38.9 | 1.37 | 91.2 | 13.7 | 52.3 | 38.9 | 1.35 | 49.3 | 51.3 |
| 3 | 96.5 | 15.2 | 55.1 | 41.4 | 1.33 | 95.5 | 14.8 | 54.0 | 41.4 | 1.31 | 49.8 | 51.8 |
| 3&6/12 | 100.8 | 16.3 | 56.6 | 43.4 | 1.30 | 99.6 | 15.9 | 55.6 | 43.9 | 1.27 | 50.0 | 52.6 |
| 4 | 103.9 | 17.3 | 57.7 | 46.2 | 1.25 | 103.4 | 16.9 | 56.9 | 46.5 | 1.22 | 50.3 | 53.6 |
| 4&6/12 | 107.2 | 18.2 | 58.9 | 48.3 | 1.22 | 107.2 | 18.2 | 58.4 | 48.8 | 1.20 | 50.5 | 55.1 |
| 5 | 110.7 | 19.5 | 59.9 | 50.8 | 1.19 | 110.5 | 19.2 | 59.2 | 51.3 | 1.15 | 50.8 | 55.9 |
| 5&6/12 | 114.3 | 20.7 | 61.2 | 53.9 | 1.15 | 114.0 | 20.6 | 60.5 | 53.6 | 1.13 | 51.1 | 56.6 |
| 6 | 117.6 | 21.9 | 62.2 | 55.4 | 1.12 | 117.6 | 22.0 | 61.7 | 55.9 | 1.10 | 51.3 | 57.2 |
| 6&6/12 | 120.7 | 23.2 | 63.0 | 57.7 | 1.09 | 120.7 | 23.4 | 62.7 | 57.9 | 1.08 | 51.6 | 57.9 |
| 7 | 123.7 | 24.6 | 64.0 | 59.7 | 1.07 | 123.7 | 24.8 | 63.7 | 59.9 | 1.06 | 52.1 | 58.4 |
| 7&6/12 | 126.7 | 26.2 | 65.0 | 61.7 | 1.05 | 126.7 | 26.5 | 64.8 | 62.0 | 1.05 | 52.3 | 59.7 |
| 8 | 129.8 | 27.7 | 65.8 | 64.0 | 1.03 | 129.8 | 28.1 | 66.0 | 63.8 | 1.04 | 52.3 | 61.0 |
| 8&6/12 | 132.6 | 29.4 | 67.1 | 65.5 | 1.02 | 132.6 | 29.9 | 67.3 | 65.3 | 1.03 | 52.6 | 61.7 |

NORMAL MEASUREMENTS BY AGE (continued)

| | MALE | | | | | FEMALE | | | | | BOTH SEXES | |
|---|---|---|---|---|---|---|---|---|---|---|---|---|
| | HEIGHT cm. | WEIGHT kg. | UPPER SEGMENT cm. | LOWER SEGMENT cm. | U/L ratio | HEIGHT cm. | WEIGHT kg. | UPPER SEGMENT cm. | LOWER SEGMENT cm. | U/L ratio | HEAD cm. | CHEST cm. |
| 9 | 135.4 | 31.1 | 68.3 | 67.1 | 1.02 | 135.4 | 31.6 | 68.3 | 67.1 | 1.02 | 52.6 | 62.2 |
| 9&6/12 | 138.2 | 33.0 | 69.1 | 69.1 | 1.00 | 138.2 | 33.5 | 69.6 | 68.6 | 1.01 | 52.8 | 63.0 |
| 10 | 141.0 | 34.9 | 70.1 | 70.9 | 0.99 | 141.0 | 35.5 | 70.6 | 70.4 | 1.00 | 52.8 | 63.8 |
| 10&6/12 | 143.3 | 36.9 | 70.9 | 72.4 | 0.98 | 144.3 | 37.8 | 72.1 | 72.1 | 1.00 | 53.1 | 65.0 |
| 11 | 145.8 | 38.9 | 72.1 | 73.7 | 0.98 | 147.6 | 40.2 | 73.4 | 74.2 | 0.99 | 53.1 | 66.3 |
| 11&6/12 | 148.6 | 41.1 | 73.4 | 75.2 | 0.98 | 150.9 | 42.9 | 75.2 | 75.7 | 0.99 | 53.3 | 67.6 |
| 12 | 151.4 | 43.3 | 74.9 | 76.5 | 0.98 | 154.2 | 45.6 | 76.7 | 77.5 | 0.99 | 53.3 | 68.6 |
| 12&6/12 | 154.4 | 45.7 | 76.5 | 77.9 | 0.98 | 157.0 | 47.9 | 78.2 | 78.7 | 0.99 | 53.6 | 68.9 |
| 13 | 157.5 | 48.0 | 77.7 | 79.8 | 0.97 | 159.5 | 50.2 | 79.8 | 79.8 | 1.00 | 53.8 | 71.1 |
| 13&6/12 | 161.3 | 51.1 | 79.5 | 81.9 | 0.97 | 161.0 | 52.4 | 80.5 | 80.5 | 1.00 | 54.1 | 72.4 |
| 14 | 164.8 | 54.1 | 81.3 | 83.6 | 0.97 | 162.8 | 54.6 | 81.8 | 81.0 | 1.01 | 54.6 | 73.7 |
| 14&6/12 | 167.9 | 57.1 | 82.8 | 85.1 | 0.97 | 163.8 | 56.3 | 82.3 | 81.5 | 1.01 | 54.9 | 75.2 |
| 15 | 171.2 | 60.1 | 84.8 | 86.4 | 0.98 | 164.8 | 57.5 | 82.8 | 82.0 | 1.01 | 55.4 | 77.0 |
| 15&6/12 | 173.2 | 62.3 | 86.1 | 87.1 | 0.99 | 165.1 | 58.4 | 83.1 | 82.0 | 1.01 | 55.4 | 77.0 |
| 16 | 175.3 | 64.5 | 87.4 | 87.9 | 0.99 | 165.6 | 59.3 | 83.3 | 82.3 | 1.01 | 55.6 | 80.5 |
| 16&6/12 | 176.0 | 65.8 | 87.6 | 88.4 | 0.99 | 165.6 | 60.0 | 83.3 | 82.3 | 1.01 | 55.9 | 82.0 |
| 17 | 176.5 | 67.1 | 87.6 | 88.6 | 0.99 | 165.6 | 60.7 | 83.3 | 82.3 | 1.01 | 55.9 | 83.8 |

GROWTH CHARTS

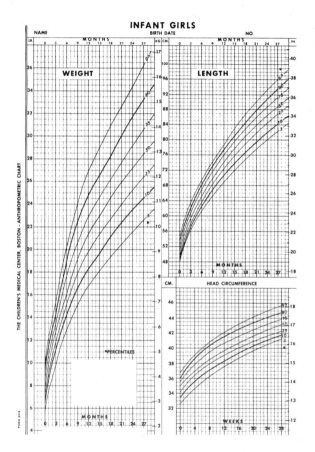

GROWTH CHARTS

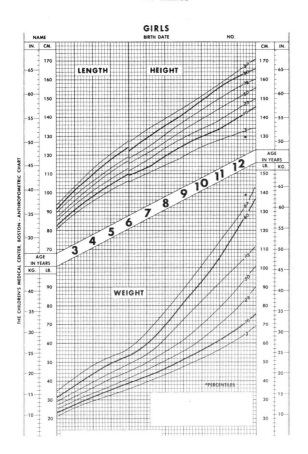

GROWTH CHARTS

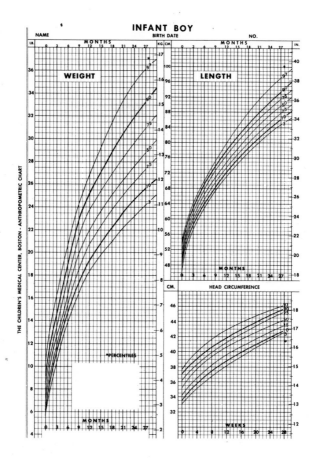

GROWTH CHARTS

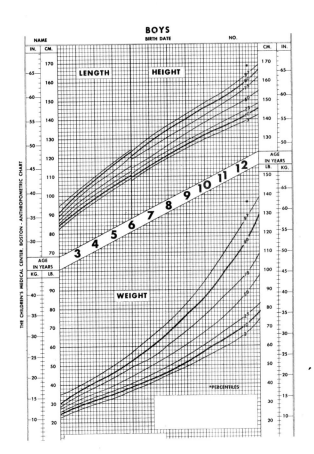

BOYS

254

HEAD CIRCUMFERENCE - GIRLS

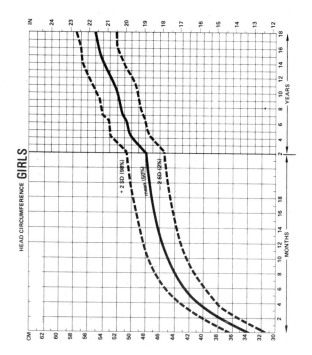

Ref: Nellhaus, G., Pediatrics 41:106, 1968

255

HEAD CIRCUMFERENCE - BOYS

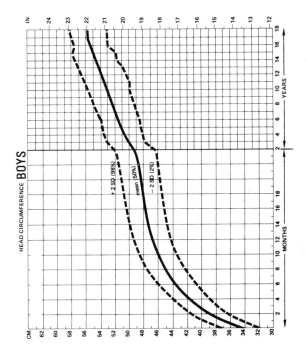

Ref: Nellhaus, G., Pediatrics <u>41</u>: 106, 1968

# INTRAUTERINE GROWTH

## Length and Weight

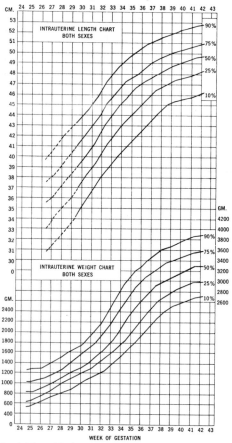

From Lubchenco, L.O., et al.: Pediatrics 37:403, 1966.

# INTRAUTERINE GROWTH

## Head Circumference and Weight/Length Ratio

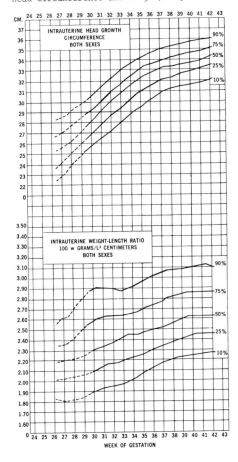

INTRAUTERINE HEAD GROWTH
CIRCUMFERENCE
BOTH SEXES

INTRAUTERINE WEIGHT-LENGTH RATIO
100 w GRAMS/L³ CENTIMETERS
BOTH SEXES

WEEK OF GESTATION

258

PREMATURE GROWTH CHART

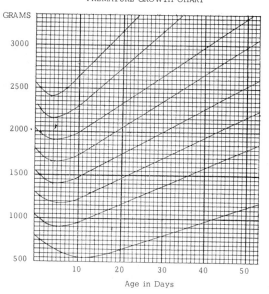

HEAD CIRCUMFERENCE/AGE CHART
FOR PREMATURES

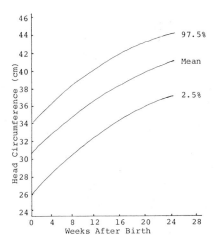

Ref: Arch. Dis. Child., 36:241, 1961.

SURFACE AREA NOMOGRAM

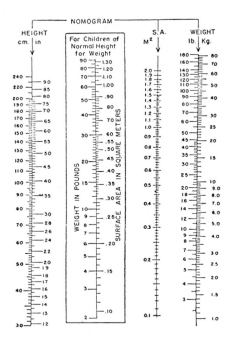

Nomogram for estimation of surface area. The surface area is indicated when a straight line which connects the height and weight levels intersects the surface area column; or if the patient is roughly of average size, from the weight alone (enclosed area). (Nomogram modified from data of E. Boyd by C. D. West.)

BONE AGE

## Age-at-Appearance Percentiles for Epiphyses and Round Bones*

| OSSIFICATION CENTERS | Boys Percentiles | | | Girls Percentiles | | |
|---|---|---|---|---|---|---|
|  | 5th | 50th | 95th | 5th | 50th | 95th |
| **Shoulder** | | | | | | |
| Head of humerus | birth | 2w | 4m | birth | 2w | 4m |
| Coronoid of scapula | birth | 2w | 4m | birth | 2w | 5m |
| Tubercle of humerus | 3m | 10m | 2y 4m | 2m | 6m | 1y 2m |
| Acromion of scapula | 12y 2m | 13y 9m | 15y 6m | 10y 4m | 11y 11m | 15y 4m |
| Accessory coronoid | 12y 9m | 14y 4m | 16y 4m | 10y 4m | 12y 3m | 14y 4m |
| **Elbow** | | | | | | |
| Capitellum | 3w | 4m | 1y 1m | 3w | 3m | 9m |
| Radial head | 3y | 5y 3m | 8y | 2y 3m | 3y 10m | 6y 3m |
| Medial epicondyle | 4y 3m | 6y 3m | 8y 5m | 2y 1m | 3y 5m | 5y 1m |
| Olecranon of ulna | 7y 9m | 9y 8m | 11y 11m | 5y 7m | 8y | 9y 11m |
| Lateral epicondyle | 9y 3m | 11y 3m | 13y 8m | 7y 2m | 9y 3m | 11y 3m |
| **Wrist** | | | | | | |
| Capitate | birth | 3m | 7m | birth | 2m | 7m |
| Hamate | 2w | 4m | 10m | birth | 2m | 7m |
| Distal radius | 6m | 1y 1m | 2y 4m | 5m | 10m | 1y 8m |
| **Hip** | | | | | | |
| Head of femur | 3w | 4m | 8m | 2w | 4m | 7m |
| Greater trochanter | 1y 11m | 3y | 4y 4m | 1y | 1y 10m | 3y |
| Os acetabulum | 11y 11m | 13y 6m | 15y 4m | 9y 7m | 11y 6m | 13y 5m |
| Iliac crest | 12y | 14y | 15y 11m | 10y 10m | 12y 9m | 15y 4m |
| Ischial tuberosity | 13y 7m | 15y 3m | 17y 1m | 11y 9m | 13y 11m | 16y |

| OSSIFICATION CENTERS | Boys Percentiles | | | Girls Percentiles | | |
|---|---|---|---|---|---|---|
| | 5th | 50th | 95th | 5th | 50th | 95th |
| **Knee** | | | | | | |
| Proximal tibia | birth | 2w | 1m | birth | birth | 2w |
| Proximal fibula | 1y 10m | 3y 6m | 5y 3m | 1y 4m | 2y 7m | 3y 11m |
| Patella | 2y 7m | 4y | 6y | 1y 6m | 2y 6m | 4y |
| Tibial tubercle | 9y 11m | 11y 10m | 13y 5m | 7y 11m | 10y 3m | 11y 10m |
| **Foot** | | | | | | |
| Cuboid | birth | 1m | 4m | birth | 3w | 2m |
| Third cuneiform | 3w | 6m | 1y 7m | birth | 3m | 1y 3m |
| Os calcis | 5y 2m | 7y 7m | 9y 7m | 3y 6m | 5y 4m | 7y 4m |

*Modified from Garn, S.M., Rohman, C.G., and Silverman, F.N.: Medical Photography 43:45, 1967.

## STANDARD ATLASES

Hand: Greulich, W.W. and Pyle, S.I.: Radiographic Atlas of Skeletal Development of the Hand and Wrist. Stanford University Press, Stanford, California, Second Edition, 1959.

Knee: Pyle, S.I. and Hoerr, N.L.: Radiographic Standard Reference for the Growing Knee. Charles C. Thomas, Springfield, Illinois, 1969.

PRIMARY OR DECIDUOUS TEETH

| | Calcification | | Eruption | | Shedding | |
|---|---|---|---|---|---|---|
| | Begins at | Complete at | Maxillary | Mandibular | Maxillary | Mandibular |
| Central incisors | 5th fetal mo. | 18-24 mos. | 6-8 mos. | 5-7 mos. | 7-8 yrs. | 6-7 yrs. |
| Lateral incisors | 5th fetal mo. | 18-24 mos. | 8-11 mos. | 7-10 mos. | 8-9 yrs. | 7-8 yrs. |
| Cuspids | 6th fetal mo. | 30-36 mos. | 16-20 mos. | 16-20 mos. | 11-12 yrs. | 9-11 yrs. |
| First molars | 5th fetal mo. | 24-30 mos. | 10-16 mos. | 10-16 mos. | 10-11 yrs. | 10-12 yrs. |
| Second molars | 6th fetal mo. | 36 mos. | 20-30 mos. | 20-30 mos. | 10-12 yrs | 11-13 yrs. |

Sexes are combined although girls tend to be slightly advanced over boys.

Averages are approximate values derived from various studies.

SECONDARY OR PERMANENT TEETH

| | Calcification | | Eruption | |
| | Begins at | Complete at | Maxillary | Mandibular |
|---|---|---|---|---|
| Central incisors | 3-4 mos. | 9-10 yrs. | 7-8 yrs. | 6-7 yrs. |
| Lateral incisors | Max., 10-12 mos.<br>Mand., 3-4 mos. | 10-11 yrs. | 8-9 yrs. | 7-8 yrs. |
| Cuspids | 4-5 mos. | 12-15 yrs. | 11-12 yrs. | 9-11 yrs. |
| First premolars | 18-21 mos. | 12-13 yrs. | 10-11 yrs. | 10-12 yrs. |
| Second premolars | 24-30 mos. | 12-14 yrs. | 10-12 yrs. | 11-13 yrs. |
| First molars | Birth | 9-10 yrs. | 6-7 yrs. | 6-7 yrs. |
| Second molars | 30-36 mos. | 14-16 yrs. | 12-13 yrs. | 12-13 yrs. |
| Third molars | Max., 7-9 yrs.<br>Mand., 8-10 yrs. | 18-25 yrs. | 17-22 yrs. | 17-22 yrs. |

Ref: Nelson, Waldo E. Textbook of Pediatrics, 1964.

NORMAL BLOOD PRESSURE VALUES AT VARIOUS AGES

| Age in Years* | Mean Systolic | Range in 95% of Normal Children | Age in Years* | Mean Diastolic | Range in 95% of Normal Children |
|---|---|---|---|---|---|
| 1/2-1 year | 90 | ±25 | 1/2 - 1 year | 61 | ±19 |
| 1 - 2 years | 96 | ±27 | 1 - 2 years | 65 | ±27 |
| 2 - 3 years | 95 | ±24 | 2 - 3 years | 61 | ±24 |
| 3 - 4 years | 99 | ±23 | 3 - 4 years | 65 | ±19 |
| 4 - 5 years | 99 | ±21 | 4 - 5 years | 65 | ±15 |
| 5 years | 94 | ±14 | 5 years | 55 | ±9 |
| 6 years | 100 | ±15 | 6 years | 56 | ±8 |
| 7 years | 102 | ±15 | 7 years | 56 | ±8 |
| 8 years | 105 | ±16 | 8 years | 57 | ±9 |
| 9 years | 107 | ±16 | 9 years | 57 | ±9 |
| 10 years | 109 | ±16 | 10 years | 58 | ±10 |
| 11 years | 111 | ±17 | 11 years | 59 | ±10 |
| 12 years | 113 | ±18 | 12 years | 59 | ±10 |
| 13 years | 115 | ±19 | 13 years | 60 | ±10 |
| 14 years | 118 | ±19 | 14 years | 61 | ±10 |
| 15 years | 121 | ±19 | 15 years | 61 | ±10 |

*Data for 1/2-5 years from Allen-Williams, G.M.: Pulse-rate and blood pressure in infancy and early childhood. Arch Dis Child. 20:125, 1945.
Data for 5-15 years from Graham, A.W.; Hines, E. A., Jr.; and Gage, R. P.: Blood pressure in children between the ages of five and sixteen years. Amer J Dis Child, 69:203, 1945.

BLOOD PRESSURE

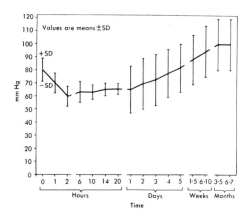

Mean systolic blood pressure in the first seven months.
The mean is plotted along with two standard deviations.
(Reproduced from Goodman, H. G., Cummings, G. R., and
Raber, M. B.: Photocell oscillometer for measuring
systolic pressure in newborn. Amer. J. Dis. Child.,
103:152, 1962.)

## RECOMMENDED DAILY DIETARY ALLOWANCES
### FOOD AND NUTRITION BOARD, NATIONAL RESEARCH COUNCIL, REVISED 1968

| Age (yrs) | Wt. (kg) | Ht. (cm) | Calories | Protein (gm) | Cal-cium (gm) | Iron (mg) | Vit. A (I.U.) | Thia-mine (mg) | Ribo-flavin (mg) | Nia-cin (mg) | Ascor-bic Acid (mg) | Vit. D (I.U.) |
|---|---|---|---|---|---|---|---|---|---|---|---|---|
| In-fant 0-1/2 | 7 | 63 | Kg x 115 | Kg x 2.0 | 0.5 | Kg x 1.0 | 1,500 | 0.4 | 0.4 | 6 | 35 | 400 |
| 1/2-1 | 9 | 72 | Kg x 100 | Kg x 1.8 | 0.6 | 15 | 1,500 | 0.5 | 0.6 | 8 | 35 | 400 |
| Chil-dren 1-3 | 13 | 87 | 1,200 | 25 | 0.8 | 15 | 2,000 | 0.6 | 0.8 | 8 | 40 | 400 |
| 3-6 | 18 | 107 | 1,500 | 30 | 0.8 | 10 | 2,500 | 0.8 | 0.8 | 11 | 40 | 400 |
| 6-9 | 26 | 126 | 2,100 | 40 | 1.0 | 10 | 3,500 | 1.1 | 1.3 | 15 | 40 | 400 |
| Boys 9-12 | 35 | 140 | 2,400 | 45 | 1.1 | 10 | 4,500 | 1.3 | 1.4 | 16 | 40 | 400 |
| 12-14 | 43 | 151 | 2,700 | 50 | 1.4 | 18 | 5,000 | 1.4 | 1.4 | 18 | 45 | 400 |
| 14-18 | 59 | 170 | 3,000 | 60 | 1.4 | 18 | 5,000 | 1.5 | 1.5 | 20 | 55 | 400 |
| Girls 9-12 | 35 | 140 | 2,200 | 50 | 1.1 | 18 | 4,500 | 1.1 | 1.3 | 15 | 40 | 400 |
| 12-14 | 44 | 154 | 2,300 | 50 | 1.3 | 18 | 5,000 | 1.2 | 1.5 | 15 | 45 | 400 |
| 14-18 | 53 | 158 | 2,300 | 55 | 1.3 | 18 | 5,000 | 1.2 | 1.5 | 15 | 50 | 400 |

## COMPOSITION OF INFANT FORMULAS

| Formula | Calories per oz. | Calories per cc. | Percentage wt/vol Protein *( ) | Fat *( ) | CHO *( ) | mEq/L Na | K | mg/L Ca | P | Ca/P ratio | mg/L Fe | Approx. Solute Load Renal (mOsm/liter) | GI |
|---|---|---|---|---|---|---|---|---|---|---|---|---|---|
| Cho-free (undiluted) | 23 | .77 | 3.60(19) | 7.00(81) | 0.04(0) | 30 | 44 | 1700 | 1260 | 1.35/1 | 16 | 260 | - |
| Cho-free with 12.8% dextrose | 20 | .67 | 1.80(11) | 3.50(49) | 6.40(40) | 15 | 22 | 850 | 630 | 1.35/1 | 8 | 130 | - |
| Cow's milk | 20 | .67 | 3.30(20) | 3.70(51) | 4.80(29) | 25 | 35 | 1240 | 950 | 1.30/1 | 1 | 220 | 270 |
| Enfamil 13** | 13 | .43 | 1.00(9) | 2.40(50) | 4.50(41) | 11 | 12 | 355 | 300 | 1.18/1 | Tr | 80 | 185 |
| Enfamil 20** | 20 | .67 | 1.50(9) | 3.70(49) | 7.00(42) | 11 | 19 | 546 | 462 | 1.18/1 | Tr | 120 | 285 |
| Enfamil 24 | 24 | .80 | 1.80(9) | 4.50(50) | 8.30(41) | 13 | 22 | 655 | 555 | 1.18/1 | 15 | 145 | 355 |
| EVM 1:1 | 20 | .67 | 3.65(20) | 4.20(51) | 5.30(29) | 28 | 39 | 1375 | 1055 | 1.30/1 | Tr | 250 | 300 |
| EVM 2:3 | 16 | .53 | 2.92(20) | 3.28(51) | 4.24(29) | 22 | 31 | 1100 | 845 | 1.30/1 | Tr | 200 | 250 |
| EVM 2:3 + 5% DM | 22 | .75 | 2.90(16) | 3.25(38) | 8.80(46) | 22 | 31 | 1100 | 845 | 1.30/1 | Tr | 200 | 300 |
| Human milk (breast) | 20 | .67 | 1.20(7) | 3.80(51) | 7.00(42) | 7 | 14 | 340 | 162 | 2.10/1 | 1.5 | 81 | - |
| Isomil | 20 | .67 | 2.00(12) | 3.60(48) | 6.80(40) | 13 | 18 | 700 | 500 | 1.40/1 | 12 | 126 | 255 |
| Lofenalac | 20 | .67 | 2.33(14) | 2.70(35) | 8.76(51) | 14 | 17 | 630 | 473 | 1.33/1 | 13 | 140 | 450 |
| Lonalac | 20 | .67 | 3.40(21) | 3.50(49) | 4.80(30) | 1.1 | 26 | 1100 | 1000 | 1.10/1 | 2 | 200 | - |
| Lytren | 9 | .28 | 0(0) | 0(0) | 7.00(100) | 25 | 25 | 80 | 155 | 0.52/1 | 0 | 106 | 540 |
| Neo-Mullsoy | 20 | .67 | 1.80(11) | 3.50(49) | 6.40(40) | 17 | 25 | 800 | 600 | 1.33/1 | 8 | 130 | - |
| Nutramigen | 20 | .67 | 2.20(13) | 2.60(35) | 8.76(52) | 14 | 17 | 630 | 473 | 1.33/1 | 13 | 140 | 460 |
| Pedialyte | 6 | .20 | 0(0) | 0(0) | 5.00(100) | 30 | 20 | 80 | 0 | --- | 0 | 80 | 400 |
| Portagen | 20 | .67 | 2.36(14) | 3.20(42) | 7.74(44) | 14 | 21 | 630 | 473 | 1.33/1 | 13 | 160 | 210 |
| Pregestimil | 20 | .67 | 2.20(13) | 2.80(36) | 8.80(51) | 14 | 17 | 630 | 473 | 1.33/1 | 13 | 140 | 640 |
| Premature formula 24 | 24 | .80 | 2.80(14) | 3.70(41) | 9.10(45) | 20 | 32 | 970 | 800 | 1.21/1 | Tr | 210 | 430 |
| Probana | 20 | .67 | 4.20(25) | 2.20(29) | 7.90(46) | 26 | 31 | 1155 | 893 | 1.29/1 | Tr | 280 | 605 |

*Percentage calories supplied by...

**Also comes with Fe (12 mg/L)

## COMPOSITION OF INFANT FORMULAS (continued)

| Formula | Calories per oz. | Calories per cc. | Percentage wt/vol Protein *( ) | Percentage wt/vol Fat *( ) | Percentage wt/vol CHO *( ) | mEq/L Na | mEq/L K | mg/L Ca | mg/L P | Ca/P ratio | mg/L Fe | Approx. Solute Load Renal GI (mOsm/liter) | |
|---|---|---|---|---|---|---|---|---|---|---|---|---|---|
| Prosobee | 20 | .67 | 2.50(15) | 3.40(45) | 6.80(40) | 18 | 19 | 788 | 525 | 1.50/1 | 13 | 160 | 250 |
| Similac Advance | 16.5 | .55 | 2.80(21) | 2.00(33) | 6.20(46) | 15 | 26 | 800 | 600 | 1.33/1 | 18 | 180 | 340 |
| Similac 13 | 13 | .43 | 1.19(11) | 2.34(48) | 4.52(41) | 10 | 15 | 450 | 360 | 1.25/1 | Tr | 90 | 185 |
| Similac 20** | 20 | .67 | 1.55(9) | 3.60(48) | 7.20(43) | 11 | 19 | 580 | 430 | 1.35/1 | Tr | 110 | 285 |
| Similac 24 | 24 | .80 | 2.20(11) | 4.30(47) | 8.50(42) | 15 | 27 | 830 | 660 | 1.26/1 | 15 | 155 | 325 |
| Similac 27 | 27 | .90 | 2.47(11) | 4.80(47) | 9.55(42) | 16 | 31 | 930 | 740 | 1.26/1 | Tr | 180 | 440 |
| Similac PM 60/40 | 20 | .67 | 1.57(9) | 3.54(47) | 7.56(44) | 7 | 15 | 400 | 200 | 2.00/1 | 12 | 105 | 250 |
| Skim milk | 10 | .33 | 3.50(40) | 0.20(5) | 4.80(55) | 26 | 34 | 1240 | 1010 | 1.23/1 | Tr | 240 | 270 |
| SMA | 20 | .67 | 1.50(9) | 3.60(48) | 7.20(43) | 7 | 14 | 420 | 312 | 1.35/1 | 12 | 105 | - |

* Percentage calories supplies by . . .
** also comes with Fe (12 mg/L)

INGREDIENTS OF INFANT FORMULAS

| Product | Protein | Fat | Carbohydrate | Comments |
|---------|---------|-----|--------------|----------|
| Casec | Soluble Calcium caseinate | Butterfat | - - - - | Protein Supplement |
| Cho-free | Soy protein isolate | Soy oil | Add 12.8% dextrose | Carbohydrate & cow-protein intolerance |
| Cow's milk | 80% casein, 20% whey | Butterfat | lactose | |
| Enfamil | Skim milk | Corn, soy, coconut oils | lactose | |
| Evaporated milk | Cow's milk | Butterfat | lactose | |
| Human milk | 40% casein, 60% whey | Human milk fat | lactose | |
| Isomil | Soy isolate & methionine | Corn, coconut oils | sucrose, dextrose maltose, dextrins corn starch | Cow protein and lactose intolerance |
| Lofenalac | Casein hydrolysate (low phenylalanine) | Corn oil | sucrose, maltose, dextrins, tapioca starch | PKU |
| Lonalac | Casein | Coconut oil | lactose | Low salt content |
| Lytren | - - - | - - - | dextrose | |
| Neo-mullsoy | Soy isolate & methionine | Soy oil | sucrose | Lactose and cow-protein intolerance |
| Nutramigen | Casein hydrolysate | Corn oil | sucrose, tapioca starch | Sensitivity to intact milk protein, lactose intolerance |
| Pedialyte | - - - | - - - | sucrose | |
| Portagen | Casein | MCT, (fractionated coconut oil) corn oil | dextrose, maltose sucrose, lactose (0.15%) | Fat malabsorption, lactose intolerance (liver disease) |

INGREDIENTS OF INFANT FORMULAS (continued)

| Product | Protein | Fat | Carbohydrates | Comments |
|---|---|---|---|---|
| Pregestimil | Casein hydrolysate | MCT, (fractionated coconut oil) corn oil | dextrose, tapioca starch (no lactose) | Readily absorbed |
| Premature formula 24 | Skim milk | Corn oil | lactose, sucrose | High protein content |
| Probana | Cow's milk & casein hydrolysate | Butterfat | lactose, banana powder, dextrose | High protein, low fat (fat malabsorption, celiac) |
| Prosobee | Soy isolate & methionine | Soy oil | sucrose, dextrose maltose, dextrins | Lactose & cow protein intolerance |
| Similac | Skim milk | Corn, soy, coconut oils | lactose | |
| Similac PM 60/40 | Skim milk & demineralized whey | Corn, coconut oils | lactose | Low salt content |
| SMA | Skim milk & demineralized whey | Corn, coconut soy oils | lactose | Low salt content |
| Vivonex | Purified amino acids | Safflower oil | glucose, oligosaccharides | Rapid absorption |

COMPARISON OF HUMAN MILK WITH COW'S MILK

COMPARISON OF HUMAN MILK WITH COW'S MILK (WHOLE AND EVAPORATED)

| | Human Milk % | Cow's Milk Whole % | Cow's Milk Evaporated % |
|---|---|---|---|
| Water | 87.0-88.0 | 83.0-88.0 | 73.0-74.0 |
| Protein | 1.0-1.5 | 3.2-4.1 | 6.8-7.0 |
| Lactalbumin | 0.7-0.8 | 0.5 | 1.1 |
| Casein | 0.4-0.5 | 3.0 | 5.7 |
| Sugar (Lactose) | 6.5-7.5 | 4.5-5.0 | 9.8-10.0 |
| Fat | 3.5-4.0 | 3.5-5.2 | 7.9-8.2 |
| (More olein and less of the volatile fatty acids) | | | |
| Minerals | 0.15-0.25 | 0.7-0.75 | 1.5-1.6 |
| Calcium | 0.034-0.045 | 0.122-0.179 | |
| Phosphorus | 0.015-0.040 | 0.090-0.196 | |
| Magnesium | 0.005-0.006 | 0.013-0.019 | |
| Sodium | 0.011-0.019 | 0.051-0.060 | |
| Potassium | 0.048-0.065 | 0.138-0.172 | |
| Chlorine | 0.035-0.043 | 0.098-0.116 | |
| Sulphur | 0.0035-0.0037 | 0.030-0.032 | |
| Iron | 0.0001 | 0.00004 | |
| Copper | 0.00003 | 0.00002 | |
| Vitamins (per 100 cc): | | | |
| A | 60-500 I.U. | 80-220 I.U.* | No loss |
| D | 0.4-10.0 I.U. | 0.3-4.41 I.U.* | No loss |
| C | 1.2-10.8 mg. | 0.9-1.4 mg* | 0.6 mg.+ |

COMPARISON OF HUMAN MILK WITH COW'S MILK (continued)

| | Human Milk % | Cow's Milk | |
| | | Whole % | Evaporated % |
|---|---|---|---|
| Thiamine | 0.002-0.036 mg. | 0.03-0.04 mg.* | 0.02-0.03 mg.+ |
| Riboflavin | 0.015-0.080 mg. | 0.010-0.26 mg.* | No loss |
| Niacin | 0.10 mg-0.20 mg.* | 0.10 mg. | |
| Reaction | Alkaline or amphoteric | Acid or amphoteric | Acid or amphoteric |
| Bacteria | None | Present | None |
| Digestion | | Less rapidly | |
| Emptying of Stomach | | Less rapidly | |
| Curd | Soft, Flocculent | Hard, large | Soft, Flocculent |
| Calories per fluid oz. | 20 | 20 | 44 |

*Values are for pasteurized milk.
Values are from Nelson - Textbook of Pediatrics, 1959.

BLOOD CHEMISTRIES

*Alkaline phosphatase:
(1 King-Armstrong unit = 7.08 milli-International
Unit (m-I.U.))

| | |
|---|---|
| Birth | 35-105 m-I.U./ml |
| 1 month-1 year | 70-250 m-I.U./ml |
| 1-3 years | 70-210 m-I.U./ml |
| 3-10 years | 70-180 m-I.U./ml |
| 10-16 years | 100-275 m-I.U./ml |

*Acid phosphatase (total):
(1 King-Armstrong unit = 1.77 milli-International
Unit (m.I.U.))

| | |
|---|---|
| Birth | 3-6 m-I.U./ml |
| 1 month-1 year | 6.5-11 m-I.U./ml |
| 1-3 years | 6.5-11 m-I.U./ml |
| 3-10 years | 3.5-9 m-I.U./ml |
| 10-16 years | 3-10 m-I.U./ml |

*Aldolase:                    <11 milliunits/ml

 Ammonia:                     <150 micrograms %
                              (Seligson Blood Ammonia)

*Amylase, serum:             <160 caraway units/100 ml

 Ascorbic acid:              over 0.3 mg%

*Bicarbonate ($CO_2$ capacity
 or combining power):        22-30 mEq/L

*Bilirubin:

| | |
|---|---|
| Cord: | up to 1.8 mg% |
| 2-4 days: | mean peak 7 mg%, range 2-12 mg% |
| After newborn period: | less than 0.8 mg% total |

*Bromsulphalein Retention:
 (at 45 minutes)

| | |
|---|---|
| Newborn: | up to 20% |
| Thereafter: | less than 5% |

*Calcium:                    9.0-11.5 mg%

*Carotene:

| | |
|---|---|
| Newborn: | 25 micrograms % |
| Thereafter: | 60-180 micrograms % |

*Chloride:                    94-106 mEq/L

*Cholesterol:                 150-275 mg%,
                              65-76% esterified

Copper:

  1 month:                    50-100 micrograms %
  1 year:                     110-175 micrograms %
  5-17 years:                 80-280 micrograms %
  Adult:                      80-180 micrograms %

*Creatine phosphokinase:      <50 milliunits/ ml

*Creatinine:                  0.7-1.5 mg%

*Fibrinogen, plasma:          200-400 mg/ml

*Glucose (fasting):           55-100 mg%

*Haptoglobin:                 1:32-1:256

Iodine, Protein Bound:

  Newborn:                    6-10.7 micrograms %
  1 week:                     9-14 micrograms %
  1-12 weeks:                 5.6-9.2 micrograms %
  3-12 months:                5.3-7.3 micrograms %
  Thereafter:                 3.5-8.0 micrograms %

Butanol extractable iodine averages 0.5 micrograms lower.

Iron:

|            | Mean Serum Fe | Total Fe Binding Capacity | Percent Saturation |
|------------|---------------|---------------------------|--------------------|
| 1 week:    | 148 micro-gm% | 262 micro-gm%             | 65                 |
| 3 months:  | 50            | 350                       | 15                 |
| 6-12 months: | 106         | 429                       | 25                 |
| 1-2 years: | 95            | 414                       | 22                 |
| 2-6 years: | 116           | 395                       | 28                 |
| 6-12 years: | 127          | 340                       | 38                 |

Ketones:                      up to 3 mg%

Lactic Acid (fasting):        up to 10 mg% if precipitated
                              STAT, otherwise, up to
                              20 mg%

*Lactic Dehydrogenase:        0-300 milliunits/ml

Lead:                          under 0.04 mg%

*Lipids:

  Total:                       450-1000 mg%
  Phospholipids:               mean 225 mg% (usually
                               slightly higher than
                               cholesterol)

*Magnesium:                    1.5-2.5 mEq/L

 Mucoproteins:
  (as tyrosine):               1.9-4.5 mg%

*pH (arterial whole            7.35-7.45 (0.03 lower in
  blood:                       venous blood)

*PCO2 (arterial):              35-45 mm Hg

*PO2 (arterial):               75-100 mm Hg

*Phenylalanine:                <3 mg%

*Phosphorus, inorganic:

  1st year:                    4-7 mg%
  1-12 years:                  5-6 mg%
  Adult:                       3-4.5 mg%

*Porcelain:                    8-20 mEq/L

*Potassium:

  0-10 days:                   up to 7 mEq/L
  Thereafter:                  3.5-5.0 mEq/L

*Proteins:

  Total:                       6-8 gm%
  Albumin:                     4.7-5.7 gm%
  Globulin:                    1.3-2.5 gm%

Proteins:    Average (Range) in Grams

| Age | Total | Albumin | Globulin | Gamma Globulin |
|---|---|---|---|---|
| Premature | 5.5 | 3.7 | 1.8 | 0.7 |
| | (4.6) | (2.5-4.5) | (1.2-2) | (0.5-0.9) |
| FT Newborn | 6.4 | 3.4 | 3.1 | 0.8 |
| | (5-7.1) | (2.5-5) | (1.2-4) | (0.7-0.9) |
| 1-3 months | 6.6 | 3.8 | 2.5 | 0.3 |
| | (4.7-7.4) | (3-4.2) | (1-3.3) | (0.1-0.5) |
| 3-12 months | 6.8 | 3.9 | 2.6 | 0.6 |
| | (5-7.5) | (2.7-5) | (2-3.8) | (0.4-1.2) |
| 1-15 years | 7.4 | 4.0 | 3.1 | 0.9 |
| | (6.5-8.6) | (3.2-5) | (2-4.4) | (0.6-1.2) |

| *Sodium | 136-145 mEq/L |
|---|---|

Tocopherol (Vitamin E):

| Premature: | 0.05-0.35 mg% |
|---|---|
| FT newborn: | 0.1-0.35 mg% |
| 2-5 months: | 0.2-0.6 mg% |
| 6-24 months: | 0.35-0.8 mg% |
| 2-12 years: | 0.55-0.9 mg% |
| Adult and breast-fed babies: | 0.6-1.1 mg% |

*Transaminases:

| SGOT | <19 milliunits/ml |
|---|---|
| SGPT | <17 milliunits/ml |

*Urea Nitrogen:  *(own)*
  Non-protein nitrogen:   6-23 mg%

*Uric Acid:   2.5-8.0 mg%

Vitamin A:   >40 micrograms %

Zinc Turbidity:

| Newborn: | less than 10 |
|---|---|
| 1-8 months: | less than 3 |
| 9-12 months: | less than 5 |
| Thereafter: | less than 8 |

*These determinations are done by The Johns Hopkins Hospital routine laboratory on serum, and the values quoted apply to their methods. Values for other determinations are taken from the literature and may not be valid for a given laboratory.

# SEROLOGY

Below are the tests that the JHH lab routinely performs.
If a desired test is not mentioned below, the lab will
send the blood to an appropriate lab elsewhere.

## Normal Values.

| | | |
|---|---|---|
| ASO | - | <1:128 |
| Anti-hyaluronidase | - | <1:200 |
| ANA | - | <1:40 |
| CRP | - | negative |
| Mono Spot Test | - | negative |
| Paratyphoid A & B | - | <1:80 |
| Proteus OX-19 | - | <1:80 |
| R.A. (Latex) | - | negative |
| Rose Test | - | titer with sensitized cells should be less than 5 times the titer with washed cells |
| Rubella | - | HAI titer |
| STS | - | negative |
| Typhoid O, H | - | <1:80 |

## All Complement Fixations Should Be Negative or <1/8:

Brucellosis
Cytomegalic Inclusion Disease
Eastern and Western Equine Encephalitis
Epidemic Typhus
Influenza Type A (F.M.I. & P.R. 8)
Influenza Type B (Lee)
Lymphocytic Choriomeningitis
Lymphogranuloma Venereum
Mumps
Psittacosis
Q Fever (American)
Rickettsial Pox
Rocky Mountain Spotted Fever
St. Louis Encephalitis
Toxoplasmosis
Tularemia

## CEREBROSPINAL FLUID

| | |
|---|---|
| Amount (obtainable by LP): | |
| Newborn: | up to 5 ml |
| Adult: | 100-150 ml |
| | |
| Initial pressure: | |
| Newborn: | 50-90 mm CSF |
| Infant: | 40-150 mm |
| Child: | 70-200 mm |
| | |
| Specific Gravity: | 1.005-1.009 |
| | |
| pH at 38°C: | 7.33-7.42 |
| | |
| Calcium: | 4.5-5.5 mg% (approximates ionized serum Ca) |
| | |
| Cell count: | |
| Newborn: | up to 25 WBC (av. 8) and up to 650 RBC/mm$^3$ |
| After 1st month: | up to 7 lymphocytes |
| | |
| Glucose: | 40-80 mg% (at least 1/2 of blood sugar) |
| | |
| Pandy (mainly globulin): | 0 (may be positive in newborn) |
| | |
| Protein (80% albumin): | |
| Ventricular: | 5-15 mg% |
| Cisternal: | 5-25 mg% |
| Lumbar: | 5-40 mg% up to 150 mg% in newborn* |
| | |
| G-O Transaminase: | 4-14 units, often about 1/2 of SGOT |

*There is too little data available on newborn CSF to define normal limits or to allow fine diagnostic distinctions.

Ref: Wyers, H.J.G., and Bakker, J.C.W.: Neederland Tijdschrift voor Kindergeneeskunde. 22:253, 1954.

IMMUNOGLOBIN LEVELS AT DIFFERENT AGES

| AGE | IgG (± 2 SD range) 100-110% Maternal Level | IgA (± 2 SD range) | IgM (± 2 SD range) Male | Female |
|---|---|---|---|---|
| Cord Blood | | 0 | 11 (0-23) | |
| 2-4 mos. | 362 (142-930) | 17 (5-64) | 44 (14-142) | 44 (16-125) |
| 5-8 mos. | 433 (250-1190) | 34 (10-87) | 62 (24-167) | 59 (50-163) |
| 9-14 mos. | 633 (322-1245) | 40 (17-94) | 80 (30-212) | 79 (29-216) |
| 15-23 mos. | 863 (466-1600) | 63 (22-178) | 81 (35-189) | 100 (44-240) |
| 2-3 yrs. | 808 (400-1620) | 71 (27-192) | 83 (41-168) | 81 (33-196) |
| 3 1/2-4 1/2 yrs. | 963 (615-1530) | 100 (42-238) | 92 (31-272) | 126 (37-425) |
| 5-6 yrs. | 976 (625-1530) | 121 (44-334) | 86 (38-197) | 86 (30-248) |

IMMUNOGLOBIN LEVELS AT DIFFERENT AGES (continued)

| AGE | IgG (± 2 SD range) | IgA (± 2 SD range) | IgM (± 2 SD range) | |
|---|---|---|---|---|
| | | | Male | Female |
| 7-8 yrs. | 1010 (615-1655) | 102 (42-288) | 73 (24-225) | 100 (35-282) |
| 9-10 yrs. | 1090 (766-1560) | 142 (43-435) | 85 (35-208) | 123 (43-348) |
| 11-12 yrs. | 1095 (727-1650) | 150 (44-508) | 73 (22-237) | 111 (41-272) |
| 13-14 yrs. | 1090 (840-1390) | 172 (59-505) | 82 (37-183) | 107 (58-196) |
| 15-16 yrs. | 1160 (879-1540) | 170 (61-420) | 93 (38-223) | 142 (75-271) |
| 17-18 | 1070 (686-1680) | 183 (80-419) | 86 (26-281) | 145 (45-463) |
| 19-21 yrs. | 964 (655-1420) | 155 (47-508) | 84 (37-191) | 123 (49-308) |
| Adult | 1044 (710-1540) | 174 (60-490) | 87 (37-204) | 104 (42-261) |

Adapted from: J. Peds. 72:276, 1968 and Ped. Clin. N. A. 18:104, 1971.

P141   200-300,000

% RBC/total vol.

% infection
68 fighters

new RBC

## HEMATOLOGY

| | Gm. Hgb. | % Hct. | WBC/mm³ | % Polys | % Retics |
|---|---|---|---|---|---|
| 1 day | 16-22* | 53-73* | 18,000 (7-35,000) | 45-85 | 2.5-6.5 |
| 1 week | 13-20* | 43-66* | 10,000 (4-20,000) | 30-50 | 0.1-4.5 |
| 1 month | 16 | 53 | 10,000 (6-18,000) | 30-50 | 0.1-1.0 |
| 3 months | 11.5 | 38 | 10,000 (6-17,000) | 30-50 | 0.7-3.0 |
| 6 months | 12 | 40 | 10,000 (6-16,000) | 30-50 | 0.7-2.3 |
| 1 year | 12 | 40 | 10,000 (6-15,000) | 30-50 | 0.6-1.7 |
| 2-6 years | 13 | 43 | 9,000 (7-13,000) | 35-55 | 0.5-1.0 |
| 7-12 years | 14 | 46 | 8,500 (5-12,000) | 40-60 | 0.5-1.0 |

Absolute eosinophil count:  100-600/mm³, average 250

*Under the age of 1 month capillary Hgb and Hct exceed venous:

    1 hour:   3.6 gm av. difference
    5 days:   2.2 gm av. difference
    3 weeks:  1.1 gm av. difference

## AVERAGE NORMAL BONE MARROW VALUES

| WBC | Normal % and Range |
|---|---|
| "Blasts" | 2.0(0.3-5.8) |
| Undiff. myelocytes (A & B) | 5.0(1.0-8.0) |
| Diff. myel. (0)-neutro | 12.0(5.0-19.0) |
| "    "    " -eosino. | 1.5(0.5-3.0) |
| "    "    " -baso. | 0.3(0-0.5) |
| Metamyelocytes - neutro. | 22.0(13.0-32.0) |
| "          -eosino. | |
| P.M.N. neutrophils | 20.0(7.0-30.0) |
| "    eosinophils | 2.0(0.5-4.0) |
| "    basophils | 0.2(0-0.7) |
| Monocytes | 2.0(0.5-5.0) |
| Lymphocytes | 10.0(3.0-17.0) |
| Plasma Cells | 0.4(0-2.0) |
| Reticulum cells & macrophages | 0.2(0.2-2.0) |
| Mitotic figures | |
| Unclassified cells | |

| RBC | |
|---|---|
| Megaloblasts | 0 |
| Pronormoblasts | 4.0(1.0-8.0) |
| Basophilic normoblasts  ) | |
| Polychromatophilic norm.) | 18.0(7.0-32.0) |
| Orthochromatic norm.    ) | |

McLEAN, HASTINGS NOMOGRAM

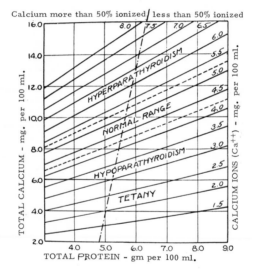

TOTAL SERUM PROTEINS VS. TOTAL SERUM SOLIDS

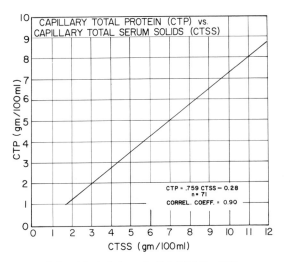

Ref: Adapted from J. Ped 71:413, 1967

UMBILICAL ARTERY AND VEIN CATHETERIZATION

Note: Shoulder-umbilical length is measured as a
perpendicular line dropped from the tip of the
shoulder to a line extended from the umbilicus.

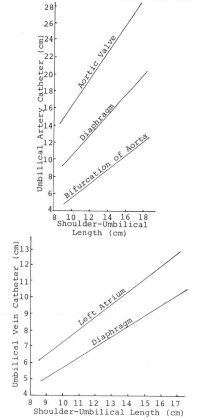

Adapted from Arch. Dis. Child. <u>41</u>: 69, 1966

## CONVERSION FORMULAS

### Weight

| Grams | Pounds |
|-------|--------|
| 454   | 1.0    |
| 1000  | 2.2    |

To change pounds to grams, multiply by 454.

To change kilograms to pounds, multiply by 2.2.

### Length

To convert inches to cms, multiply by 2.54.

### Temperature

To convert centigrade to Fahrenheit:
$(9/5 \times \text{temperature}) + 32$
To convert Fahrenheit to centigrade:
$(\text{Temperature} - 32) \times 5/9$

## TEMPERATURE EQUIVALENTS

| Centigrade | Fahrenheit | Centigrade | Fahrenheit |
|------------|------------|------------|------------|
| 34.0 | 93.2  | 38.6 | 101.4 |
| 34.2 | 93.6  | 38.8 | 101.8 |
| 34.4 | 93.9  | 39.0 | 102.2 |
| 34.6 | 94.3  | 39.2 | 102.5 |
| 34.8 | 94.6  | 39.4 | 102.9 |
| 35.0 | 95.0  | 39.6 | 103.2 |
| 35.2 | 95.4  | 39.8 | 103.6 |
| 35.4 | 95.7  | 40.0 | 104.0 |
| 35.6 | 96.1  | 40.2 | 104.3 |
| 35.8 | 96.4  | 40.4 | 104.7 |
| 36.0 | 96.8  | 40.6 | 105.1 |
| 36.2 | 97.1  | 40.8 | 105.4 |
| 36.4 | 97.5  | 41.0 | 105.8 |
| 36.6 | 97.8  | 41.2 | 106.1 |
| 36.8 | 98.2  | 41.4 | 106.5 |
| 37.0 | 98.6  | 41.6 | 106.8 |
| 37.2 | 98.9  | 41.8 | 107.2 |
| 37.4 | 99.3  | 42.0 | 107.6 |
| 37.6 | 99.6  | 42.2 | 108.0 |
| 37.8 | 100.0 | 42.4 | 108.3 |
| 38.0 | 100.4 | 42.6 | 108.7 |
| 38.2 | 100.7 | 42.8 | 109.0 |
| 38.4 | 101.1 | 43.0 | 109.4 |

CONVERSION OF POUNDS AND OUNCES TO GRAMS

| Ounces | 1 lb. | 2 lb. | 3 lb. | 4 lb. | 5 lb. | 6 lb. | 7 lb. | 8 lb. |
|---|---|---|---|---|---|---|---|---|
| | | | | GRAMS | | | | |
| 0 | 454 | 907 | 1,361 | 1,814 | 2,268 | 2,722 | 3,175 | 3,629 |
| 1 | 482 | 936 | 1,389 | 1,843 | 2,296 | 2,750 | 3,204 | 3,657 |
| 2 | 510 | 964 | 1,418 | 1,871 | 2,325 | 2,778 | 3,232 | 3,686 |
| 3 | 539 | 992 | 1,446 | 1,899 | 2,353 | 2,807 | 3,260 | 3,714 |
| 4 | 567 | 1,021 | 1,474 | 1,928 | 2,381 | 2,835 | 3,289 | 3,742 |
| 5 | 595 | 1,049 | 1,503 | 1,956 | 2,410 | 2,863 | 3,317 | 3,771 |
| 6 | 624 | 1,077 | 1,531 | 1,985 | 2,438 | 2,892 | 3,345 | 3,799 |
| 7 | 652 | 1,106 | 1,559 | 2,013 | 2,466 | 2,920 | 3,374 | 3,827 |
| 8 | 680 | 1,134 | 1,588 | 2,041 | 2,495 | 2,948 | 3,402 | 3,856 |
| 9 | 709 | 1,162 | 1,616 | 2,070 | 2,523 | 2,977 | 3,430 | 3,884 |
| 10 | 737 | 1,191 | 1,644 | 2,098 | 2,552 | 3,005 | 3,459 | 3,912 |
| 11 | 765 | 1,219 | 1,673 | 2,126 | 2,580 | 3,033 | 3,487 | 3,941 |
| 12 | 794 | 1,247 | 1,701 | 2,155 | 2,608 | 3,062 | 3,515 | 3,969 |
| 13 | 822 | 1,276 | 1,729 | 2,183 | 2,637 | 3,090 | 3,544 | 3,997 |
| 14 | 851 | 1,304 | 1,758 | 2,211 | 2,665 | 3,119 | 3,572 | 4,026 |
| 15 | 879 | 1,332 | 1,786 | 2,240 | 2,693 | 3,147 | 3,600 | 4,054 |

# INDEX